W9-BYV-197

How to Survive and Maybe Even Love Nursing School!

about the author

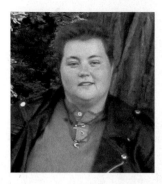

A Rubert Scholar and 1998 honors graduate of MCP-Hahnemann University School of Nursing in Philadelphia, Pa., Kelli S. Dunham, RN, is now in that school's MSN program. She works as a staff nurse at MCP-Hahnemann School of Nursing Health Center, a nurse-managed primary care center in North Philadelphia. In addition, she is a professional writer specializing in humor, and currently has a biweekly column in a Philadelphia magazine, *Au Courant*.

Kelli has worked as a hospice volunteer among AIDS patients in Haiti, as a night manager at a shelter for the homeless in Norristown, Pa., as a legal assistant and translator for Florida Rural Legal Services, and as a caseworker for Project H.O.M.E. In-Community in Philadelphia. This is her first book.

How to Survive and Maybe Even Love Nursing School!

A Guide for Students by Students

By Kelli S. Dunham, RN, BSN

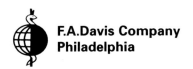

F.A.Davis Company
Philadelphia

F. A. Davis Company
1915 Arch Street
Philadelphia, PA 19103
www.fadavis.com

Copyright © 2001 by F. A. Davis Company

Copyright © by F. A. Davis Company. All rights reserved. This book is protected by copyright. No part of it may be reproduced, stored in a retrieval system, or transmitted in any form or by any means, electronic, mechanical, photocopying, recording, or otherwise, without written permission from the publisher.

Printed in the United States of America

Last digit indicates print number: 10 9 8 7 6 5 4 3 2 1
Acquisitions Editor: Lisa A Biello
Developmental Editor: Melanie Freely
Production Editor: Jessica Howie Martin
Cover Designer: Louis J. Forgione

As new scientific information becomes available through basic and clinical research, recommended treatments and drug therapies undergo changes. The author and publisher have done everything possible to make this book accurate, up to date, and in accord with accepted standards at the time of publication. The author, editors, and publisher are not responsible for errors or omissions or for consequences from application of the book, and make no warranty, expressed or implied, in regard to the contents of the book. Any practice described in this book should be applied by the reader in accordance with professional standards of care used in regard to the unique circumstances that may apply in each situation. The reader is advised always to check product information (package inserts) for changes and new information regarding dose and contraindications before administering any drug. Caution is especially urged when using new or infrequently ordered drugs.

Library of Congress Cataloging-in-Publication Data

Dunham, Kelli S.
    How to survive and maybe even love nursing school! : a guide for students by students/ by Kelli S. Dunham.
        p. cm.
    Includes bibliographical references and index.
    ISBN 0-8036-0799-7 (pbk.)
    1. Nursing—Study and teaching. 2. Nursing students—Psychology. 3. Nursing students—Anecdotes. I. Title.
RT73.D79 2001
610.73'071'1—dc21

2001017087

Authorization to photocopy items for internal or personal use, or the internal or personal use of specific clients, is granted by F. A. Davis Company for users registered with the Copyright Clearance Center (CCC) Transactional Reporting Service, provided that the fee of $.10 per copy is paid directly to CCC, 222 Rosewood Drive, Danvers, MA 01923. For those organizations that have been granted a photocopy license by CCC, a separate system of payment has been arranged. The fee code for users of the Transactional Reporting Service is: 8036-0799/01 + $.10.

In December 1995, Liz Walz worked for a luxury hotel, pampering those our society calls "VIPs." In December 1999, Liz participated in the Plowshares versus Depleted Uranium project, making our planet a little safer for all people.

Liz doesn't like to be considered a hero, and she most assuredly doesn't want to be called a saint. "We all have spiritual challenges every day," she says. "Nothing we do will ever be big enough, and nothing we do is too small."

But in a world where violence goes unnoticed in its omnipresence, every nonviolent choice is heroic and every act of resistance is sacred.

This book is dedicated to Liz, with thanks.

Kelli S. Dunham

To Nancy, Eric, Emily, and Sparky

— They know why.

– Peter H. Johnson

foreword

I think we can all agree that preparing for, attending, and successfully completing a rigorous program of study in nursing school is a challenge that will not soon be forgotten by anyone who bravely undertakes it. It's probably one of the most difficult things you'll do in your life, but it promises to be a highly rewarding experience if you approach it methodically, energetically, and in a focused manner. And—as this book shows—by lightening up just a bit.

In *How To Survive and Maybe Even Love Nursing School!*, Kelli Dunham, a registered nurse who is currently a student in an MSN program, has gathered a rich collection of ideas and facts that will help you prepare for and survive this positively life-changing experience. Kelli shows that if you use a focused approach, you'll be able to find the one nursing school that's right for you, and once you've found it, you'll have a richer and more fulfilling educational experience.

Nursing students (and prospective nursing students) need practical tips, resources, and information to help them succeed in school, and Kelli Dunham's first-person account provides these with an immediacy that you don't get elsewhere. What's more, she delivers with a humorous, breezy style enriched by numerous personal stories contributed by many of the 300 students and faculty members she interviewed for the book.

How To Survive and Maybe Even Love Nursing School! gives hard-hitting advice on choosing and getting into a nursing school, finances and financial aid, the importance of time (and life) management, dealing with information overload and stress, forming study habits that streamline the learning experience, study skills and resources, test taking, being a nontraditional (older, gay/lesbian, male) student, handling clinical rotations, preparing for and taking the NCLEX, licensure, issues and trends in nursing, and finding and landing that perfect job. Two helpful appendices give further advice on using computers in nursing school and using humor in healing. The chapters and appendices offer up-to-the minute resource lists of additional readings and useful Web sites, which Kelli has personally reviewed.

I urge all prospective and current nursing students to read this informative, helpful, and interesting book, as it contains a wealth of information that will enrich many aspects of your learning journey. Kelli has broken new ground in explicating the unique nursing school experience.

After reading the many first-person anecdotes from nursing students in *How To Survive and Maybe Even Love Nursing School!*, I can't resist offering a handy hint of my own for a nightly study routine. The night after your first class, read over your notes from that day. The second night, read your notes from days 1 and 2; the third night, read your notes from days 1, 2, and 3. And so on. This sounds like a tremendous commitment of time and energy, but it's so easy because, as you read over your notes, you begin to integrate them and memorize them. Each succeeding night, you'll need less and less time to read your earlier notes. And by the end of the semester, you've just about memorized every word. It worked for me!

Going to nursing school can be a hectic and frustrating experience, but take time occasionally to pause and reflect on the reasons why you chose nursing as your life's work. Among these, I hope, is a strong desire to serve others—or else I doubt many of you will be able to persevere when the going gets tough. Serving as an instrument through which healing can occur is truly a blessing. As an aspiring nurse, you have announced to the world that you feel you have the courage to do the often difficult work of healing. If you find on your journey that you are going through a dark night of the soul, remember that nursing offers both the caregiver and the patient the wonderful opportunity to be inspired with the healing breath of God! That, dear friends, is very, very precious.

Paula Schneider, RN, MPH, editor of Healing Hearts *(Vista Publications), a collection of true and inspiring stories written by nurses from all over the world about special patients who have touched their lives forever.*

introduction

Who am I and why am I writing this book?

Before I started nursing school, I lived in Haiti, Oklahoma City, Southeast Ohio, Miami, and Harlem. I worked as a hospice volunteer, legal assistant/interpreter for an organization assisting Haitian refugees, and night manager at a homeless shelter. I was even a Roman Catholic nun in training for 11 arduous months. After 10 relatively happy but exhausting years, I realized I wanted a career instead of just a succession of jobs.

After a substantial amount of navel gazing and procrastinating, in 1996 I started nursing school at MCP-Hahnemann University and graduated with my Associate Degree in Nursing in May 1998. On September 23, 1998, I received my RN license. I completed my BSN in May, 2000, and I am now a student in an MSN public health nursing program. I also work as a staff nurse in a nurse-managed health center located within a medically underserved area of North Philadelphia.

I will readily admit that my reasons for becoming a nurse are half altruistic and half pragmatic. It's true that I want to work with other people in order to enable them to have long, happy, and fulfilling lives, but I also want to have a long, happy, and fulfilling life myself. I chose nursing because I felt that it would provide opportunities for both. I suppose, at age 32, it's a little early for me to say if I qualify as having a "long" life, but so far, becoming a nurse has been all I thought it would be, and more.

It was the influence of five friends who all have RN after their names that ultimately helped me make the final decision to start nursing school. These friends are experienced nurses, and it is their advice that got me through school. They displayed admirable patience when I'd call them the night before clinical and ask them—"just one more time"—about the procedure for suctioning a tracheostomy tube. They lent me everything from stethoscopes to textbooks. They dispensed freely their time, advice, and words of support. They had walked the same road I was walking and were able to point out the beautiful scenery (and the potential detours) along the way. Not everyone has the benefit of exposure to nurses like these when they are in school. My hope is that this book will be a resource that, like my five friends, makes the path through nursing school more productive and enjoyable for those who take it.

This book is meant to be a comprehensive guide to nursing school, so I've covered everything from completing your first admission application to getting your first job. In addition, because this book is written from a student's perspective (over 300 students provided input), I have been able to deal realistically with the nitty-gritty details of life as a nursing student. Are you worried about getting "grossed out" by something at clinical? Read Chapter 7 to see how other nursing students have handled this possibility. Do you always fall asleep when you read your textbooks? See Chapter 4 for tips on handling an overwhelming reading load. Bewildered or disgusted by the conditions you see in hospitals where you do your clinical rotations? Check out Chapter 9 to learn ways to advocate for a better system.

Another feature that developed out of my nursing school experience is the "Profiles in Nursing" scattered throughout the text. I can vividly remember mornings when I would sit on the side of my bed at 5:15 AM. I knew I needed to get up and get dressed for clinical, but I would nevertheless spend several minutes staring blankly at my feet, wondering what on earth I was doing in nursing school. I've included these profiles for those moments when students need an inspiration infusion. Some of the individuals profiled have held traditional nursing positions in hospitals and branched out, so to speak, while others work in outpatient facilities, community nonprofit agencies, or even cyberspace. What they all have in common is a love for nursing and a desire to help the nursing profession fulfill its potential.

So you've decided to go to nursing school

If you're very far at all along in your nursing school career, probably at least one person has said to you: "Nursing school? Nursing school? Now why on earth would you want to do that?!" This is annoying when the person is a significant other or friend, discouraging when it's a parent, but downright demoralizing when it's a nurse.

It's true, many people find nursing school stressful. You may wake up one night in the middle of your third semester and realize that you have again started sucking your thumb when you sleep, a habit you thought you gave up for good in the first grade.

It's true that many people find nursing school unbelievably time consuming. You may start to wonder what you did with all your free time when you were only raising children and working 50 hours a week.

It's true that there will be days when you will feel sleep deprived and nutrition deprived and sunlight deprived and fun deprived and self-esteem deprived.

But there will also be days when things will start to come together. There will be a moment when pharmacology and physiology will do a happy dance together in your brain, or when microbiology will seem like the living science that it is, instead of just boring culture plates and senseless diagrams depicting virus replication. There will be days when you can bring comfort to a patient and, in so doing, comfort yourself.

It may feel daunting today, but you can do it. The path may seem long, rocky, and arduous, but there is an "RN" at the end.

You *can* do it. Let's go.

Kelli S. Dunham

acknowledgments

"Men anpil, chay pa lou"

"Many hands make the load light"

— Itaitian proverb

Although it is my name that is on the spine, I am acutely aware that this book is very much a group effort. "Thank you" seems like a rather anemic response to the generosity with which many people have supported this project.

I have been both lucky and delighted to work with Alan Sorkowitz, Pete Johnson, and Lisa Biello at F. A. Davis Company. As the man with the idea for this book and the ultimate responsibility for making sure the project stayed on track, Alan was a faithful guide from the first e-mail we exchanged. Lisa has also been a champion since her first connection with the project. In fact, everyone with whom I've had contact at F. A. Davis has been consistently courteous and helpful. This has made working with F. A. Davis, something I already considered an honor, a pleasure as well.

Pete Johnson has had the difficult task of being both the illustrator for this project and the developmental editor trying to coach a first-time author into creating a book. Pete is high-energy, detail-oriented, and persistent; in short, he is ideal for his responsibilities. I am very grateful for his help and even more grateful I didn't have his job!

Over 300 nursing students, nurse educators, new grads, and staff nurses—many of whom I know only through e-mail correspondence—provided valuable input for this book. You'll meet some of them in these pages. Their questions, stories, tips, and advice have made this book what it is, as has the input of the many student and faculty reviewers who have shared their time and thoughts. In addition, the wisdom of Becca Hover, co-chair of the GenderPAC Board of Directors, greatly helped shape Chapter 6.

acknowledgments

Closer to home, my experience at MCP-Hahnemann University School of Nursing has been such that to adequately document how supportive the folks there have been would require a book in itself. I especially appreciate the support of the William E. and Theresa M. Rubert Memorial Trust throughout my undergraduate school years.

My co-workers at MCP-Hahnemann School of Nursing Health Center have taught me what teamwork can accomplish and changed the way I think about problem solving. It is a rare work environment that combines cramped space, hard work, and serious fun. I have the blessing of working in such a place. In addition, my co-workers have been flexible and generous when I was dealing with deadlines for this project. This book could not have been written without their help.

Dorothy Day said, "We have all known the long loneliness and the answer is love, and that love comes in community." It is the rare day when I am not reminded of how extraordinary my community is:

Maura ("AMC") Kelly is my business manager and best friend. In addition to taking care of the more left-brained side of my writing projects, during the time I was writing this book she has acted as a jester, gentle pest, and much-needed distraction. The loose ends of this project were tied up at Maura's apartment, and her only requirement was that I not sing the "fundamenta-friendependability" song after 3 AM. She is quite a friend.

My local family (Beth, Jeff, Viola, and Wesley) has also contributed to this book. My sister Beth has been a comfort with her willingness to pretend that 5 AM is a perfectly reasonable time to leave for the beach. This book has been nothing if not time consuming, and now that it's done, I owe my niece Viola and my nephew Wesley more than a few hours of playing the Dinosaur at the Bottom of the Stairs Game. This is one debt I am looking forward to paying off.

My chosen family, most specifically the "Philadelphia Tyke March" gang, has been, as always, a positive support through

acknowledgments

this process. I am proud to say that even if we don't succeed in changing the world, we have a great time trying. Hooray for strong women in comfortable shoes!

Jen Pour and Andrea Szyper, my apartment-mates during the writing of this book, in addition to always being there with a word of encouragement, have both been patient with the paper chaos that not-so-occasionally crept out from under my office door and into our common space.

I am grateful to Colleen O'Connell of *Au Courant,* who not only believes that I am talented, but also reminds me of it whenever she has a chance. A 10-minute phone conversation with Colleen can help me stay motivated for weeks. Everyone should have such a substantive cheerleader on their side.

Sometimes to go forward, you have to look back. When I didn't have the courage, Urvashi Bhagat, Linda Cohen, Cassendre Xavier and the folks of the Sanctuary community lent me theirs. With their guidance and assurance I am starting to believe that, indeed, the truth is like a second chance.

Finally, I want to recognize five nurses—John Ackerman, Rose Anderson, Mary Beth Appel, Julianna Berrigan, and Laura Coe. All these individuals, at different periods of my life, in one way or another, said "You can do it, Kelli. Go to nursing school." Well, guess what? They were right! I could do it, and I did. For this, and for the example of caring they set, they have earned my sincere thanks and boundless respect.

K.S.D.

reviewers

We express our appreciation to these individuals, nursing students and faculty, who helped make this book possible through serving as reviewers and contributing their advice.

Renee Bender, RN
Kent State University
Kent, Ohio

Debbie Crosby, BSN
BSN, East Carolina University
Greenville, North Carolina

Tommy Duvall, RN, BSN, EMT
Texas Tech University Health Sciences Center School of Nursing
Lubbock, Texas

Daniel Greene, RN, ASN
Three Rivers Community College
Norwich, Connecticut

Judith K. Hovey, PhDc, MSN, RN
Assistant Professor
Oakland University School of Nursing
Rochester, Minnesota

Sandra Joyce, AD
Surry Community College
Dobson, North Carolina

Terrica Preast, BSN
Lewis-Clark State College
Lewiston, Idaho

Grace Saylor, RN, MSN
Nursing Instructor
York Technical College/USCL
Rock Hill, South Carolina

reviewers

Louise Strauser, BA, AASN
Arkansas State University
State University, Arkansas

Melody Ward, AD, LPN
Kent State University East Liverpool Campus
East Liverpool, Ohio

And we also thank the following reviewers, whose current degrees and affiliations could not be obtained at press time:

Janet Henselder
Melville, New York

Wayne Wheeler
Petersburg, VA

table of contents

▪ Chapter 3

Yes, You Can Avoid: Role
Confusion Related to
Juggling Multiple Tasks...53

▪ Chapter 4

Yes, You Can Avoid: Impaired
Memory Related to
Information Overload...69

Chapter 5

Yes, You Can Avoid: Anxiety
Related to a Life Built Around
Multiple-Choice Tests...99

■ Chapter 6

■ Chapter 7

Chapter 8

Chapter 9

■ Chapter 10

Yes, You Can Avoid: Sleep
Pattern Disturbance Related
to Occupational Worries...207

■ Appendix A

▪ Appendix B

▪ Index...265

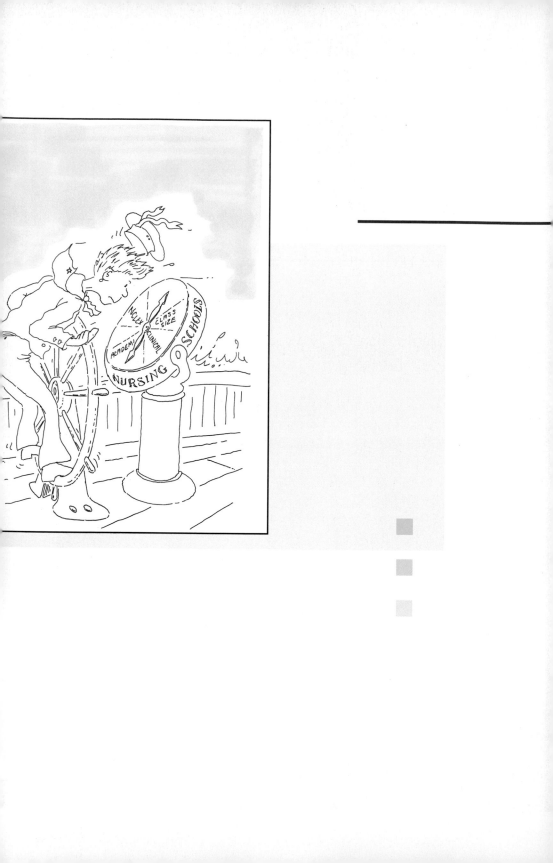

CHAPTER **1**

Yes, You Can Avoid: Confusion, Acute, Related to Multiple Choices

" students speak

"As an older student I had two main considerations. The first was the quality of education (could it get me through boards?) The second was the time it would take me to get a license and get a job. That's what steered me away from a diploma school—I didn't have the time to devote to the kind of regime they required."

— **Stan Brown, AD student, Georgia**

"I never considered anything but a diploma program and, now that it is all said and done, I'm glad. I wanted clinical time, and lots of it. I have done more IMs, hung more IVs, and cleaned up more messes than any of my friends who went to other schools."

— **R. Ledorn, diploma graduate, Florida**

> "Why would anyone want to go to school for any-
> thing less than a BSN? You'll end up having to go
> back anyway. I've learned so much from my classes,
> I can hardly imagine working as a nurse without
> them!"
>
> — **R.E., BSN student, Michigan**

If you haven't already encountered the AD-versus-BSN-versus-
diploma school debate (a.k.a. the "entry level to practice" controversy), you will. I think of it as the *Family Feud* of nursing, and it provides an interesting (if rather involved) sociological debate about the
status of nursing as a profession.

It's also pretty confusing. Have you ever tried to explain to someone
who's not familiar with the health sciences why there are three different ways to become a registered nurse? It's not easy. The dialogue
could go something like this:

> *(The scene is at a party, and Polly Patience, nursing student,
> is chatting with a new acquaintance.)*
>
> **Polly:** "So, after I finished my first year of nursing school—"
>
> **Acquaintance (interrupting):** "Oh, hey, you must go to Our
> Lady of Thunder Hospital downtown! My mother's great-aunt's
> sister graduated from there. I hear their uniforms are really
> scary!"
>
> **Polly:** "Oh, I don't go there. I go to Big Name University."
>
> **Acquaintance (scratching head):** "Big Name University. I
> didn't even know they were a hospital."
>
> **Polly:** "They aren't."
>
> **Acquaintance (looking rather frightened):** "Sheesh, well,
> I would hate to have you taking care of me if I were sick!"

(Turns away, muttering to herself) "Good grief . . . a nurse who's never been to a hospital!"

Polly: "No, wait, you *see* I do my clinical education at a couple of different hospitals. I go to a university that has a 4-year program."

Third person (joining in): "Oh, yeah, there's a nursing program at the community college I go to. But why does it take you guys 4 years to get a 2-year degree?"

Polly: "Well, it's *not* a 2-year degree. It's a bachelor of science in nursing and—"

Acquaintance: "So the people who graduate from community college aren't really registered nurses?"

Polly: "Oh, no, they are, but—"

Third person: "Hey, and what about the people who go to hospital schools? They aren't registered nurses?"

Polly: "No—I mean, yes, they are—I mean—"

(Polly's listeners walk away, shaking their heads in bewilderment. Polly didn't even get to the part about diploma, associate degree, and bachelor's degree graduates all taking the same licensure test!)

I approach this entire issue of entry level to practice with great trepidation, because whatever I say, someone—possibly many people—will express a very strong opinion about it. It's been discussed, argued about (and probably cried over) for years, so I'm not going to settle the matter once and for all in this chapter. I found it very telling that one of my early reviewers begged me not to "beat the dead AD-versus-BSN horse," and I'm inclined to think she has a point. (Note: That's a cliché—no horses were harmed in the writing of this book.)

This entry-level issue comes up on just about every nursing-related e-mail discussion group I participate in. Sometimes the exchanges are cordial and friendly, and sometimes they're borderline rude. They typically start by explaining the philosophical underpinnings of each participant's argument but end up with each person swapping hospital horror stories of how they encountered an AD/Diploma/BSN graduate who couldn't flush an I.V., write a decent care plan, communicate effectively with a patient, or whatever.

Choosing a program that fits your career objectives

Trying to "prove" what the entry level to practice should be by relating personal stories does not make a lot of sense. After all, we've all heard about incredibly talented nurses who've graduated from the tiniest diploma programs in the most pitiful hospitals, and we know of others who couldn't tell a Hoyer patient lift from a horseshoe who've graduated from respected programs in the most prestigious universities.

Perhaps a more important issue than "What nursing program is right for everyone?" is "What nursing program is right for you?" When I started interviewing students and new graduates for this book, I found that almost half didn't even consider entry level to practice as an issue when they were considering a program. They simply went ahead and chose a school with a good reputation that would work with their budget, schedule, and academic resources.

Sara Searcy, who attends Darton College in Albany, Georgia, is one example. "I always knew in the back of my mind that I wanted to be a nurse," Sara said. "The school I go to only offers an AD option, so I will transfer after becoming an RN if I want to go further. I may go for a BSN, an MSN, or both after becoming an RN. I am just going to play it by ear. Or I may work for a while and then go back to school."

Jill Hall, a nursing student in California, replied similarly, "Local junior colleges offered economical programs very close to home. Returning to school after 20 years, I was intimidated by anything bigger. I have grown since then, but

I'm glad I made the choice because I need to get out and get a job as soon as possible. But I would love to get a BSN and MSN one day." K.L, a BSN student in Wisconsin said she found "that there was a really good BSN program at a university 10 blocks from my house. Attending school there makes perfect sense!"

Perhaps if many of us were able to say, "Oh, goodness me, I have unlimited time and money and the freedom to pick up my two suitcases, a stethoscope, and my (low-maintenance) cat Fluffy and move anywhere to pursue my RN," then this discussion might be more practical. But most of us are limited in some way by our time and our responsibilities in deciding whether or not we want to move to Snowsville in northern Montana just because that's the best nursing school in the region.

Of course there are differences between programs and advantages and disadvantages of each route to the RN. I have included quotes from students about the most commonly named pros and cons and a short description of each type of program in *Students' thoughts about the programs they chose.* Although diploma school enrollments have been declining for the last 20 years, a fair number of diploma schools still exist, so I am including them here. However, students choosing diploma programs should be aware that diploma schools are quickly disappearing and may not be a viable option in the future.

As for how your degree affects your career plans, it varies even within geographic areas and specialties. Judy Reishtein, a nurse educator at Wilkes University in Wilkes-Barre, Pennsylvania, said she advises students to plan to get a BS degree. "It is required for certain positions (managerial, home health, and others) and by certain agencies," she says. "I used to tell potential students in my area who were worried about the cost to go for their AD, get licensed and get a job, and then use their tuition reimbursement benefits to pay for their RN to BS program. This option is drying up, however, as health-care agencies limit or cut tuition reimbursements."

Ann B. Fives, a nursing educator with 25 years' experience who is now affiliated with Raritan Valley Community College in New Jersey, suggests that the choice of a program should be an individual one. "It should depend on the student, their age, their financial situation, and long-term plans. For the student just graduating from high school and who has financial support from parents, I strongly advise the BSN program either as a commuter student or live-away. For the newly divorced mom who's trying to support her children, manage a home, and attend school, I advise the ADN spread out over 3 to 4

Students' thoughts about the programs they chose

PROGRAM	PROS	CONS
Diploma • Usually 3-year program • Located in a hospital, sometimes in conjunction with a community college • Prepares nurses for staff positions in hospitals and other inpatient facilities	"The diploma school in my area is very inexpensive." "I know from high school that I am the type of student who needs a lot of one-on-one time. I heard that hospital schools offer that." "We have lots of clinical time. I'm quite comfortable on the hospital floor now."	"I sometimes feel that other nurses look down on us—like we are part of a dinosaur-age system." "It's hard to work during school because you spend so much time at clinical." "It's like we're living in a fishbowl because we spend so much time around the other students!"
Associate Degree (AD) • Usually 2-year program • Usually located in a community college • Prepares nurses for staff positions in hospitals and other inpatient facilities	"Convenience—the community college I attend is 10 minutes' walk from my front door." "I already have a promise of a job when I graduate and they will pay 100% of my BSN courses. It's like getting 4 years of education for the price of 2."	"I'm afraid I won't be able to get a job anyplace else but a nursing home." "Now I have to go back to school to get my BSN. Ugh! Sometimes I wonder if it would have been easier to do it all at once."
Bachelor of science (BSN) in nursing • Usually 4- to 5-year program • Located in colleges and universities • Prepares nurses for positions in both inpatient and community settings	"It's easier to compete for a job—there are a million AD programs in my city and not that many places to work." "I'm ready to start graduate school anytime. Anytime I get the courage, that is!"	"I'm in debt up to my ears!" "I'm a sophomore and getting tired of theory classes. I just want to see a patient!"

years. I typically tell these students to take all related prerequisite courses before entering the clinical nursing portion." Melody Ward, an AD grad from Ohio adds, "[the need to] spread the curriculum out for the single mother is very important. I witnessed many students trying to compress the curriculum into the proposed 2-year program, many carrying 20 credit hours a semester; many either became overwhelmed and dropped out or lost financial assistance due to a declining grade-point average."

The logical conclusion is to consider carefully how much you can spend in time and money. Consider what you need from a program and also what you want. Then, get as much education as you can afford.

Choosing a school

" a former student speaks

"I took a very indirect route to becoming a nurse. For as long as I can remember, I always wanted to be one. I started in a 4-year program, but didn't like the school. For my second year, I transferred to a pre-nursing program knowing I would have to transfer again for years 3 and 4. I went to a very large, prestigious university for year 3. Thought I had it made. I didn't adapt to such a large school very well; there were so many distractions. I finished my third year there, but not in nursing. I returned home and went to community college. I was much more focused there, with small classes and relatively small clinical groups, and I flourished. So, after 5 years of school I had an associate degree. I always knew I would continue, and I did when the time was right, and I graduated summa cum laude while working full time and having a family. My point is—know the school well before you go. The large, prestigious university was very impersonal and too big for me to focus. It may have a great name, but that doesn't matter if it doesn't work for you! The community college I thought I was too good for turned out to be the best education money could buy and was not nearly as expensive as the other schools."

— Pat Reilly, RN, nurse-educator, Easton (Pennsyl- vania) Hospital Education Service

Okay, so now you have some idea of what type of programs you'd like to investigate. What next? First, you'll probably want to check out one of the more comprehensive guides to nursing schools so you can have a somewhat complete list of schools that are practical options for you. (See the Resources section at the end of this chapter.) After you've called or written for some prospectuses and admission packages, you can narrow the field a bit by doing some preliminary research about each school. Ask a high school guidance counselor (if there's one handy), pester your friends who are in nursing school already, surf the Web, and go to school recruitment fairs.

What should you be looking for? In general, you want a place where you can get the education that's best for you. The emphasis is on the YOU . . . not your mom, your uncle, or your spouse. You're looking for a school that meets your needs, and you know best what those needs are. In the words of Dr. Rosalee Seymour, a 30-year nursing education veteran at East Tennessee State University: "Look for FIT, FIT, FIT. If it does not fit you, look elsewhere. Fit can be social, political, financial, cultural, educational, or all these and more."

For some students this fit is obvious. "Choosing my school was not complicated," said Jodi Hancock, a BSN student in Washington State. "It is best in the state, and it's close to my home." Some students might look for a school that will grant them credit for past courses; others might want a school with flexible clinical scheduling; and still others may seek a school that's noted for its positive community involvement. Remember, when choosing a school, according to Sandra Wolf, MSN student and nurse-manager, "Nothing is laid in stone. Be a consumer. Have high expectations of a program. Education is expensive, so ultimately, you must really want this."

Choosing a school size

Some students find that the size of a school is an important factor in their choice. This was true for Stan Brown: "I happened by chance to live within 30 miles of a school of nursing with the highest first-attempt pass rate for boards in the state (91 percent to 96 percent for the past 10 years). Also, it is a small school and the instructors really get to know and care about the students. There is a real sense of community among the staff, students, and their families. One of the advantages of a small school is its intimacy." He adds, "I'm tickled about the whole thing."

Pat Reilly, a nurse-educator whom we heard from earlier, agrees: "In my experience, some of the superacademic schools have so many students that the beginning nursing student gets lost in the shuffle. I also strongly recommend small- to moderate-sized schools. I hate being in a huge lecture hall with 125 nursing students."

Larger schools may appeal to students for a variety of reasons. Some students may feel suffocated by the closeness of a smaller school. In addition, larger schools often have greater physical resources (such as more extensive library collections or a swimming pool) and may be able to provide greater access to certain opportunities, like participating in research or being involved in intercollegiate athletics.

Yet another option is to choose a regional campus of a large university, which can provide you with the advantages of a bigger school (name recognition of school by employers, access to facilities) with the atmosphere of a smaller campus.

What to look for academically

The first two academic indicators you'll want to check out are whether the school is accredited by the National League for Nursing and what the school's National Council Licensure Examination (NCLEX) pass rate is. When you ask for the NCLEX pass-rate figures, make sure they cover a 5- to 10-year period. After all, you don't want to spend several years of your life and treasure attending a school that might not provide the proper education you need to get your license. But remember that NCLEX pass rates are only one indicator of a program's academic excellence. For example, the University of Dokawatchie, located in your state's capital, may admit only the most brilliant students, who might pass the NCLEX if they spent 2 or 4 years playing Ultimate Frisbee on the moon instead of studying. Your local community college may have a more open admissions policy, admitting students who need extra tutoring or more structured environments to make it through school. The two schools might have very dissimilar pass rates, but you'd have to look at other factors to accurately judge the quality of their academic offerings.

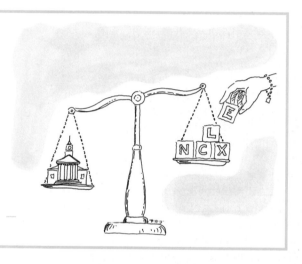

One factor that affects a school's academic quality is class size. Make sure you inquire about faculty-to-student ratios for both classroom and clinical instruction. Also ask about the typical class sizes for both prerequisite and nursing courses. Smaller size usually means more individual attention and can be helpful at any stage in school, but it is not essential in prerequisite courses and classroom nursing courses. It's more important in clinical rotations, however, because so much of clinical teaching is one-on-one with your instructor. The more students in your clinical group, the more you will be competing for the instructor's time and attention.

Ask if the school requires its faculty to practice, which can tip you off to how clinically current the instruction will be. This is paramount for clinical instructors, but it's also important for those mostly involved in classroom teaching. It's advantageous to learn the history of nursing from someone who's lived the history of nursing, but it's not so advantageous if your instructor hasn't kept clinically current and starts lecturing *ad lib* about safety precautions to take when administering ether (yes, it happened at my school).

Don't forget to check into the school's general education classes, which can make a big difference in the quality of your nursing school experience. For example, I took an anatomy and physiology course during my first college experience some years before I entered nursing school. I didn't recall a single thing from that class except a strong dislike for the smell of pickled fetal pigs. Because my original anatomy and physiology class was so old, I had to retake it in nursing school. I groaned and moaned about this at first, but I was very lucky: the class was team taught by three individuals who were *extremely* enthusiastic about their subject matter. All three had earned doctorates and all were phenomenal at explaining complicated physiological processes. Whenever I need to recall information about the effect of different electrolyte imbalances on the heart, I can close my eyes and see Dr. Kennedy flailing his arms about wildly as he demonstrated how " . . . the sodium rushes *into* the cardiac cells [flailing] and the potassium rushes *out.*" The class greatly increased my understanding of pathophysiology, and I would have really missed out if I had been permitted to settle for my original anatomy and physiology class.

What to look for clinically

First, determine whether the school provides enough clinical rotation time. Next, find out whether there are enough varied clinical placements and whether you will be placed on units where you will get hands-on experience without being made to do so much "scut work" that you won't have time to learn. It's good to learn how to stay on a schedule and how to take care of the needs of several patients, but if someone is always telling you to make up a bed for a new admission whenever there is a chance to try a new procedure, you will ultimately miss out on some valuable experiences. This probably is not something the school admissions office is going to share with you, so be prepared to ask a current student about this if you make a campus visit.

Try to find out whether or not the clinical instructors will be very familiar with the units where your rotations will take place. This can be helpful or troublesome for students. Some students say that having instructors who were too "chummy" with the nurses on the clinical unit made it hard for the instructors to be objective if there was a staff-student conflict. I have experienced this problem myself. However, I've also been grateful at times for an instructor who knew her way around enough to be able to help locate the linen closet if I couldn't find a staff nurse and needed to change a bed in a hurry.

What to look for socially

If you're a commuting student, you may think the school's social climate doesn't matter to you. But, like it or not, you will have social interaction with your classmates. It's the nature of nursing school. Of course, if you're going to be living on campus, the social climate becomes more important. If you're a new grandmother and you don't want to eat lunch every day with teenagers who just got their braces taken off and are discussing the latest issue of *Tiger Beat*, you should inquire about the age range of the students.

In addition, if you're a male student or if you're a member of a racial minority or a person with a same-sex or bisexual orientation, you may want to make a decision based at least partly on the diversity of the student body. (For more about this topic, see Chapters 6 and 7.) Of course, if a school is perfect for you in other ways, you might be able to rely on support from your family and friends if the student body is not as diverse as you would like. But because all nursing schools are not created equal when it comes to realizing that all nursing students are not created equal, it doesn't hurt to check things out in advance.

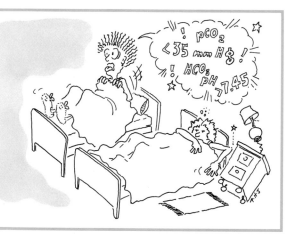

If you're staying on campus and want a roommate, ask if you can request a fellow student nurse for a roommate. There are pros and cons to this. On the pro side: A nursing school classmate can be a ready-made study partner and is likely to appreciate that the evening before clinical is not a great time for an all-night Jell-O Pit Twister Marathon. He or she will understand what a "Code Brown" is and why you grind your teeth in your sleep and wake up screaming, "It must be respiratory alkalosis!" on the night before a big exam.

Don't forget to consider how intense you are about your own work. There's probably a U.S. government study establishing a per-dorm-room quota for super-type-A-study-all-day-and-all-night nursing students, and I would be very surprised if it's any more than "one." If you know that you tend to be a grind, it might be nice to have an art history major around who makes you take a break and go visit the museums on Sunday afternoons instead of reviewing the bones of the inner ear for the umpteenth time. A non-nursing school roommate will also remind you that projectile vomiting isn't a subject that most people like to discuss at meals. This is something you and your nursing school buddies might well forget.

The risk, however, no matter what your roommate's major, is that a random turn of the Roommate Whool of Fate may pair you with someone you simply cannot stand, and the stress of nursing school combined with living with someone you don't like will probably get to both of you very quickly.

Making the most of your campus visit

If you live in the same area as the nursing schools you are considering, you will probably visit campuses at least once to complete paperwork and the like. There are many benefits to spending more time on the campus than the interval needed to dash in and drop off a recommendation before a holiday weekend.

"I definitely recommend visiting the various campuses you're interested in," said Victoria Hunter, a nursing student in Ontario, Canada. "There are so many different choices to make that an important influence on your decision will be the reaction to the campus where you will be spending the next years. Programs can be nearly identical, but your personal response to the atmosphere of the school can help you decide where you will be most comfortable and happy."

To learn more about the school's academic offerings, Deborah L. Roush, a nursing educator at Valdosta State University in Georgia, suggests "interviewing faculty, and students in and out of your major, as well as hanging out in the library and computer labs to get a feel for the learning environment. Sit in on a class or two if the instructor does not object. Look at the technology used to teach and support learning."

Take a guided tour of the school, but don't let your research stop there. Aside from soaking up the general atmosphere, there is plenty of information you can obtain with a little private detective work. Talk with at least one current student, especially one who is not leading tours. The school is generally going to have its best, brightest, and most satisfied customers out front. Maybe every student at the school does have an IQ of 170 and performs independent cellular research in their spare time, but you'll never know until you ask. Sandy

Wolf has another suggestion for self-directed sleuthing: "Make sure you notice the looks on the faces of the students and teachers."

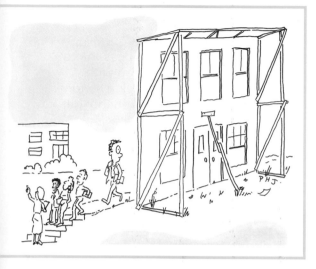

While you're at it, look at the school's physical resources. A beautiful campus does not a nursing school make. However, if you are going to be spending a lot of time on that campus and you love the sight of duck ponds and waterfalls, then by all means make that a factor in your choice of school.

You'll also want to check out the availability of computer labs, supervised nursing skill labs, and the quality of the offerings at the library. Also check how far the school is from the sites where you will be doing your clinical. This is particularly important if you will be relying on public transportation, rides from good-hearted fellow students, or your own two feet to get you there.

Finally, if you are going to be living on campus, check how close the school is to shopping, groceries, laundry, churches, and recreational opportunities. When the time comes to celebrate passing your blood pressure return demonstration, you aren't going to want to take three subways, a bus, and a dogsled to the nearest place to get a bite to eat.

Online options

If attending school, even as a commuter student, presents a hardship to you, you may want to consider taking online classes. Many schools have extensive Internet-based educational offerings. Online courses are sometimes compared to the correspondence courses of old, but the best Web courses are completely dissimilar. For example, when I was living in Haiti, I tried to take a Shakespeare class by correspondence. It required me to complete a series of very dry, uninspired assignments, and I found I couldn't finish it no matter how hard I tried. I even forced myself to carry around a copy of the textbook in my backpack every day as a motivator until I finished it. More than 10 years later, I still haven't finished that course, although I long ago stopped carrying the book around. On the other hand, I recently took a Principles of Health Promotion class offered via the Web for my RN to BSN program. It was tough and demanding, but I learned a great deal because it provided greater interaction and quicker feedback than I got in the traditional paper-based correspondence class. Not to mention that I finished it in less than a decade!

The advantages to taking online courses are obvious. For starters, you can participate in class discussions while wearing your pajamas, and you can fit your school schedule to your schedule instead of the other way around. But there are also some drawbacks. In an online class you can't see nonverbal cues during discussions, and some material may be more difficult to grasp without the benefit of classroom structure. Web courses can work for you, however, if you are a self-directed learner. For more information about online school options, see Appendix A, "Computers as a Helping Hand Through Nursing School."

Getting in

a student speaks

"I am so sick of forms! Application forms! Reference forms! Forms for financial aid! Is nursing school going to require as much paperwork as getting into nursing school?"

— G. W., AD student, Pennsylvania

After you get all the school information in the mail but before you put pen to paper, take the time to organize your efforts. Compile a fact file of information on your achievements, activities, academic background, and work experience so you can make sure you provide uniform information on each application. (Hint: You can use this file later if your self-esteem starts to fail halfway through nursing school and to prepare your resume when you graduate.)

Filling out those %#×!! forms

Applications are time consuming, annoying, redundant, and discouraging. Sadly, Internet or no Internet, they are still the only means of letting a nursing school know that you are interested in their program. I know I don't have to remind you that the application should go out neat and clean with answers in black ink or neatly typed. Photocopy the forms before you start filling them out, so that when your pet ferret zips by and spills your 64-ounce soda on your application, there will be no cause for ferreticide because you can pull out your duplicate form and use that. It's also a good idea to use the extra copies for practice before you send out the final draft, and make sure you put away the application for a day before mailing it so you can look at it with a fresh eye and catch any errors.

Many nursing schools require an essay or personal statement with their applications. If you can use this to communicate some knowledge of what nursing entails and show that you have put some thought into the decision to become a nurse, then at the very least you'll tip off the admissions committee that you are a serious applicant. If you know an alumnus of the school, it wouldn't hurt to ask for some tips. If you're really stuck, go to your local supersized bookstore, buy some overpriced coffee, and cruise their college and reference shelves. They will usually have several decent books that can provide ideas for application essays. (One suggested title is included in the Resources section in this chapter.)

When you're choosing people to write your recommendations, pay close attention to what the school is requesting. Don't have your childhood friends, relatives, or pets recommend you unless for some bizarre reason the school specifically asks for such. Make sure the person filling out the form can speak to your abilities in the areas of critical thinking, leadership, and science. Also, it doesn't hurt to slip them a list of the great things you've done and the awards and honors you've received. Sure, you want their responses to sound spontaneous, but they can't be expected to produce from memory an annotated list of all of your wonderful attributes.

Of course, the traditional etiquette you've learned about courting the people who are taking the time to write recommendations goes a long way. Don't forget to thank them—and don't forget to provide the stamp! And by the way, I know from personal experience that recommendations look better if you don't get them from the reference writer and then leave them crammed in the bottom of your bookbag for a month before you send them.

Handling interviews

The simplest way to ace an interview is to be well prepared. As MSN student Diane Langton suggests, "Reflect upon what your goals are, and how you plan to meet your goals. Think about what any obstacles may be and how you plan to tackle them. Also know your strengths and your weaknesses." To that I would add: buy a navy-blue suit (take a trip to the thrift store if need be) and wear it.

Nervousness can be a formidable foe in interviews, making it hard for us to present our best selves. However, it helps to remember that the interviewer is probably at least a little nervous, too. The person on the other side of that desk was hired to make sure the school offers the greatest opportunities to the best students who will also make the best nurses. That's not an easy task. Keep that in mind and the experience might not seem so scary. Perhaps there are some sadistic interviewers out there who just want to see you sweat, but would you really want to go to that kind of school anyway?

Remember, the interview is not only about the school evaluating you, but about you evaluating the school. Only one of the schools I applied to required an interview, and the interviewer spent 10 minutes of our time together speaking ill of the other schools I had applied to. When I made my final decision, the interviewer's unprofessional behavior was a significant factor in my deciding not to attend the school she worked for. The way the interviewer treats you can provide a clue as to how the school treats students in general. If you are kept waiting for a long time, if the tone of the questions or the interview itself is adversarial, or if there seems to be a lot of disorganization or confusion in the interview process, this may raise a red flag that says "keep looking."

Transferring credits

Surprisingly, of all the students I talked to for this book, none had any problems transferring their credits. This may say more about the good planning skills of nursing students (since most of the transfers were preplanned) than about the ease (or lack thereof) with which nursing school credits can be shuffled back and forth from one school to another.

Prerequisite classes, such as English, are the most easily transferable classes. However, it is a good idea to keep the syllabi and basic course information for each class you take, in case you later decide to transfer and the school you are going to questions the course. It is not unheard of for schools with 4-year bachelor's programs to categorically refuse to grant transfer credit for science classes, such as anatomy and physiology or chemistry, that were taken at a community college. It is always good to inquire ahead, and get the information in writing if possible, before taking any classes you hope to transfer into the school where you will take your main nursing courses.

Transferring nursing classes can be difficult. Some schools will grant credit for a similar-level course (such as Nursing 101) in the same type of program, especially if the program the credits are coming from is a known entity to the program that is receiving the credits. However, a number of schools do not accept any transferred nursing classes unless they have a pre-existing agreement with the originating school. Other schools require students to petition for courses to be accepted in lieu of other courses. The petition often must include verification of acceptable completion as well as a copy of the course syllabus describing objectives, clinical experience, and lecture topics.

If you are going to an AD program and plan on getting your BSN, ask the AD school about any *articulation agreements* they have with schools with RN to BSN programs. While you would think that an RN to BSN program would automatically accept credits a student obtained while working on their RN, this is not always the case. An articulation agreement ensures that the core classes you take toward your RN will be counted as equivalent classes in the RN to BSN program, saving you time and money and heartache later on.

Some students report difficulty in transferring credits from diploma schools. One way to decrease the risk of transfer credit being denied for courses you take at a diploma school is to choose a school that has a cooperative agreement with a community college. Many diploma schools now have these agreements, which result in graduates being granted an associate's degree from the community college and a diploma in nursing from the diploma school.

Counting the cost

" a student speaks

"I was never in debt until I went to nursing school, a fact of which I am very very proud. Now I owe over $8000. It's a little depressing, but I know there is a difference between good debt and bad debt. I owe a lot of money now, but it doesn't begin to compare with the education I have."
— **D. D., AD student, Pennsylvania**

Discovering the real costs of attendance

Nursing school tuition is not cheap, but the costs of nursing school go way beyond the cost of tuition. Most nursing schools assess many additional fees, not all of which are well advertised, so they can come along when you least expect, and can least afford, them. "I was very surprised by the costs of attendance like lab fees, uniforms, etc. It is amazing the fees they can come up with! I think they have someone thinking of new fees every year," said Jessica Wheeler, a BSN student from Connecticut. If you can, avoid sticker shock by asking the bursar's office for a complete fee list when you go to register, and make sure you include fees when comparing school costs.

Another significant first-year expense is outfitting yourself for clinical. Some schools require students to have supplemental malpractice insurance, which often has to be obtained from a specified vendor. Some rather reasonable schools allow you to wear commercially available scrubs as a uniform. You can shop around, mail order, or get hand-me-downs from other students to save some cash. At my school we were required to buy our pants, a smock top, name pin, shirt, lab coat, and goggles from the company that had a contract with the school. The bill was way over $300, and the quality of what we got was very poor. If I had known how flimsy the products were, I would have balked. Moral: Do some independent research before you buy school equipment.

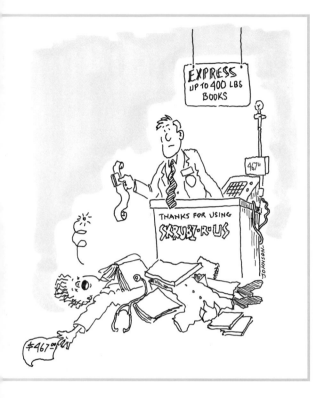

In addition to costs of basic equipment for clinical rotations, students sometimes find that they need to spend money on a computer so that they can write papers and care plans at home. When you inquire about resources available at the school, make sure you ask about the availability of 24-hour computer labs. If you are able to arrange for child care, this may be a more viable financial option than buying a computer of your own. If you do decide to purchase a computer for school, ask at the computer lab or library about computer and software discounts that may be available for students.

Aside from direct costs, being in school can put a dent in your finances in other ways. Some students told me they spent over $250 on photocopies alone during a 2-year program. In addition, if there are times when you are going to be studying instead of working, you'll need to figure in that loss of income as part of what going to school will cost you.

This is where commuting time becomes a significant cost factor. Time spent commuting is time wasted because it can't be used very easily for studying and (unless you have a rather innovative job) can't be used to earn money either. When you consider such things as the extra costs of baby-sitters, lunches, and gas for and wear and tear on your car, a community college located half a county away from you might end up being more expensive than a 4-year program right across the road. Moral: Get all the information and do the math.

Think about: government financial aid

To help you meet the costs of your nursing education, the federal and state governments dispense many forms of financial aid. Some, such as Pell grants, are outright gifts from your Uncle Sam, but Uncle has some others, such as Stafford and Perkins loans, that you have to pay back. Each of the states has financial aid programs, too. The key to getting any or all of these forms of financial help is something called the Free Application for Federal Student Aid, or FAFSA. The accent is on "federal," but many states use this document as a starting point as well. The FAFSA is about 8 pages long and can either be filed electronically through the federal Department of Education's Web site (see the Resources section at the end of this chapter) or by using the paper form—which you can either download and print directly from the federal Web site as a PDF document with Acrobat Reader—or pick one up from your school's financial aid office. The paper form will remind you of the achievement tests you took in grade school, because you have to fill in lots of teeny-weeny circles and boxes with a number-2 pencil. Unlike the Iowa Tests of Basic Skills, however, the FAFSA asks all sorts of personal questions, like what your income is, what assets you have, and much more. The cool trick about the FAFSA is that if you don't change your address between school years, the Feds will send you a renewal application the next year with most of the information already filled out for you. All you have to do is check it for accuracy and send it back in.

After your FAFSA is processed, you will receive by return mail a very important piece of paper called the Student Aid Report (SAR). Make sure you open it as soon as you get it and correct any errors you find, because the SAR is the magical document that will help determine what government financial aid you will get.

At this point, individual schools have their own procedures, so check with your school's financial aid office. The most common next step is taken by the school, which sends you a letter outlining the anticipated financial aid you will receive. This offer may not be the final word on how much aid you will receive (especially if your financial situation changes drastically after you apply for aid), but it can be useful for comparing offers from different schools.

Think about: nongovernmental financial aid

If you are not eligible for governmental assistance (for example, if you're an independent student who's been working for several years, or a traditional-age student with two working parents who own their home) and you can't pay for school on your own, don't give up hope of ever seeing the inside of a nursing school. There are several nongovernmental sources that can help.

One very common form of nongovernmental assistance is employee tuition reimbursement. If you can get it, this setup is almost ideal. What could be better than your boss paying so you can go to school free? This is a common perk for hospital employees, but it is becoming less so with downsizing and budget cuts. Even if you work at the zoo or for the circus, make sure to ask around your workplace about help with tuition. Even if there is no plan set in stone, perhaps your boss will feel some sympathy and make a personal grant to your school fund.

Nursing organizations are another source of scholarships for nursing students. The National Student Nurses Association (NSNA) awards scholarships to both members and nonmembers, and most state NSNA chapters also offer scholarships. The National League for Nursing, in addition to sponsoring its own scholarships, distributes a reference guide to scholarships for nursing students. Addresses for both these organizations' Web sites are found in the Resources section of this chapter.

Don't forget to check out some of the online scholarship searching options listed at the end of the chapter. If you do even a 30-second scan of these sites, you will realize that there are scholarships for everything. Do you have hazel eyes? A tattoo of a dolphin on your left shoulder? Was your paternal great-grandfather a conscientious objector during the Civil War? There may well be a scholarship for you.

In addition, the school you are applying to may have its own scholarship program. Ask at the financial aid office about this, but also ask directly at the school of nursing, too, since there may be scholarships that only nursing students are eligible for and that the financial aid office may forget to tell you about.

Finally, ask, ask, ask. Ask everyone you know if they have heard of any local scholarships. Work it into conversations at your kids' Little League games, e-mail all your friends (and some of your enemies), and, in general, make a nuisance of yourself. Don't be shy—it's for a good cause!

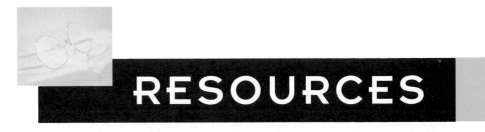

RESOURCES

Books

Georges, Christopher. (1995) *100 Successful College Application Essays.* New York: Mentor Books.

This book provides examples of unique college essays and gives suggestions for writing your own. It's easy to read and comprehensive.

Leider, Anna, and Leider, Robert (2000). *Don't Miss Out: The Ambitious Student's Guide to Financial Aid.* Alexandria, VA: Octameron Associates.

This is an annual publication with tons of references and lots of details. Check their Web site at *www.Octameron.com.*

Longacre, Doris (1980). *Living More with Less.* Scottsdale, PA: Herald Press.

This is a classic about simple (read: cheap) living, as exemplified by the Christian tradition of the Mennonite Church. Longacre includes lots of information on keeping down expenses while saving the earth and making it better for all its inhabitants. There are loads of practical hints, which make for interesting reading even if you can't imagine doing them yourself. It includes sections on clothes, homes, transportation and travel, celebrations, recipes, eating together, and the philosophical underpinnings of simple living.

Online bookstores

A number of online college bookstores have popped up on the Web recently, and this is just a somewhat representative sample. Some great deals can be had at these sites, but always comparison-shop before you buy, since prices (and shipping and handling charges) can be quite variable.

(Tip: Make sure the book you're ordering is the *same edition* as the book your instructor is using!) Try these three sites:

FATBRAIN

www.fatbrain.com

This is an online professional bookstore with a searchable database. Categories are Computing & Internet, Business, Science & Math, and General Interest. Choose: Science & Math > Life Sciences > Medicine > Nursing. The site provides Web-secure online shopping.

TEXTBOOKS.COM

www. textbooks.com

This is just what it sounds like: online searching and ordering of textbooks on all topics, not just nursing. It offers Web-secure online shopping. The site features new and used books, and it also has a guaranteed buy-back policy for books you purchase through their site (they even pick up the postage!).

Web sites

THE DOLLAR STRETCHER

www.stretcher.com

This is an easy-to-use, quick-loading, and very comprehensive site with lots of time- and money-saving tips. You can sign up for a money-saving newsletter, find recipes, and read about how to avoid consumer scams, reduce credit card debt, and even build your own log cabin.

PETERSON'S COLLEGE GUIDES

www.petersons.com

Peterson's of the Peterson's College Guides maintains this site. There is a wealth of information available on this site: a handy e-application feature, ways to compare colleges and college costs, and (no shock here) a link to their bookstore, where you can buy Peterson titles. They also have a separate but related Web site called *collegequest.com.* After you answer a series of questions to register, there's a very simple, easy-to-read guide to financial aid that covers federal, state, and college-based programs. It includes a calculator for estimating family contributions.

SAVVY STUDENT

www.savvystudent.com

This site contains all sorts of money-saving tips; it's geared toward the traditional-age student and leans heavily on the obvious for content ("Eating out is much more expensive than cooking in.") It is nonetheless a useful site, with cheap recipes and online coupons.

STUDENT ADVANTAGE

www.studentadvantage.com

This is a very large student-oriented site that includes everything from stories on health to career and dating and relationships to money and travel and tips on time management. It's clearly meant for the traditional-age student, but I recommend it for nontraditional-age students who are trying to figure out what their younger counterparts are talking about. It also has a nifty "Student Advantage Card" (you can either buy one for $20 or get one free by signing up for a calling card), which gives you discounts at several national chains as well as local merchants. Although the deals can be quite good, check around your area to make sure there are plenty of merchants who take the card; this depends largely on how many colleges are in the region.

Organizations

FASTWEB: FREE SCHOLARSHIP AND COLLEGE SEARCHES, AND FINANCIAL AID TOOLS

www.fastweb.com

Provides free, customizable searching for college and scholarship information. Basically, you enter information about yourself and they tell you what's out there. It's quick and easy and they'll update you by e-mail of any new promising scholarships.

NATIONAL STUDENT NURSES' ASSOCIATION

www.nsna.org

You can download and print applications for NSNA scholarships from this site. Some scholarships are reserved for members only, but many can be given to any eligible nursing student. You will need Adobe Acrobat Reader on your computer to access the documents. (Acrobat Reader can be downloaded for free from *www. adobe. com*.)

OFFICE OF STUDENT FINANCIAL ASSISTANCE, U. S. DEPARTMENT OF EDUCATION

http://www.fafsa.ed.gov/

You can download and print out the FAFSA forms here as well as a comprehensive student guide to financial aid. (You will need an Adobe Acrobat Reader, but if you don't have it, this site contains a link to download it.) You can also obtain the federal Title IV School Codes that you need if you're going to fill out the paper FAFSA.

CHAPTER 2

Yes, You Can Avoid: Powerlessness Related to Excessive Stress

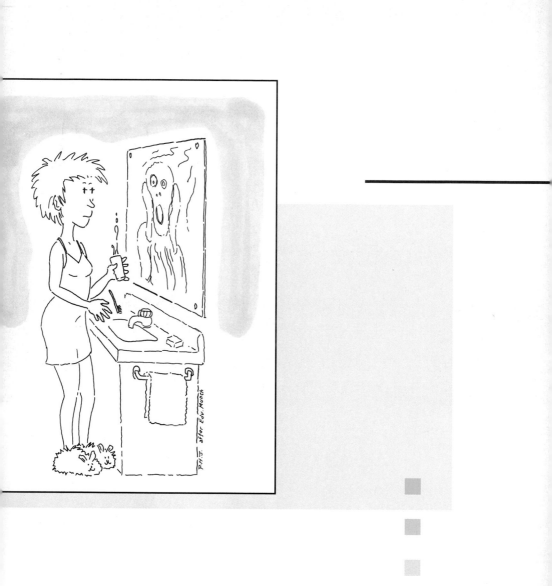

CHAPTER **2**

Yes, You Can Avoid: Powerlessness Related to Excessive Stress

" students speak

"I have been through hell and back with nursing
school, starting in one awful program and transferring to another. I have cried a million tears and had
a million anxiety attacks. I am now a senior nursing
student and am very burnt. I was in the skills lab
the other day practicing my skills and I was able to
spot all the students going into Nursing I. They were
all so excited and fresh. I am burnt beyond a crisp
and so are my classmates."
— **M.P., BSN student, Illinois**

"I have been on both sides now, from LPN to AD to
BSN to MSN. Everyone needs to lighten up, laugh a
little more, relax, and enjoy the learning. Help each
other. Trust your instincts. Savor the insights. Drink

margaritas together at the beginning of the semester instead of only at the end. Keep nursing special.
Take the messages slung around in the philosophy
classes back to the trenches. Take the practicality
and humanism of the trenches back to the classroom
and use the learning to make care better. Oh, yeah,
don't forget, 'Bs' get degrees!!"
— Sandra Wolf, MSN student, Wisconsin

Defining the problem

I was about halfway through my first semester of nursing school
when I began snapping at my friends, having trouble sleeping at
night, and mainlining chocolate as a mood stabilizer—in other
words, stressing out. I was shocked by my reaction. I had lived in
Haiti through 3 bloody military *coups d' etats,* and survived 2 years
as a nun-in-training. How could I be stressed out by simply attending
nursing school? I felt like Viane Frye, a recent graduate from an AD
program in Florida, who told me: "I anticipated the academic challenges (I have tons of school including time spent in a PhD program),
but they were nothing compared to the emotional stressors."

What makes nursing school so stressful? The students I surveyed
gave many answers, but they all agreed on one major stressor. As
Craig Moore, a student from New Zealand, put it: "Nursing school
stress is so different because if you make stuff up, you are potentially risking others' lives."

In retrospect, this makes perfect sense. When I tried my hand at college
the first time, I was an English major. I'm not saying it wasn't ever difficult or that I never ground my teeth in frustration at some school-
related headache, but the pressure I felt to achieve in the English program was somewhat mitigated because it was mostly internal. The
consequences of not being able to interpret the symbolism in a Shake-

spearean sonnet or to diagram a sentence with three dependent clauses are nothing compared with the consequences of not recognizing an order written for a freakishly high dose of digoxin or forgetting how to position a patient who is 1 day post-op after a hip replacement.

Even students accustomed to working in other health-care fields find that the complex demands of nursing school can be overwhelming. Nursing student Stan Brown worked as an EMT and emergency room technician before starting his first semester. Still, he found that "nursing school stress is different from run-of-the-mill life stress . . . because the instructors are asking (nay, insisting) that you stretch yourself in ways that you may not be accustomed to stretching. You are asked to think in an entirely different way, to coalesce static rote- and verse-memorized fact with subjective theory. You also have to utilize generalized principles with underlying caring behaviors and develop an individualized plan. All of this while keeping up with a rainforest's worth of paperwork, under the eye of a watchful practitioner who has the power to snuff out your dream like a candle in a windstorm."

Unfortunately, the "run-of-the-mill" stress that Stan talks about doesn't go away when we start nursing school. When you combine life stress and school stress, things can get difficult very quickly.

Taking control

So we know that excessive stress is bad stuff, and we know nursing school provides plenty of it. Is there anything average students can do to keep from turning into a quivering, stressed-out amebic mass before they can put the "RN" after their name?

The first thing to do is to put the stress in as positive a frame as possible, which of course is considerably easier said than done. It helps to remember that reasonable stress is helpful; we all need some stress in our life, or we would probably never get out of bed.

The second general suggestion is to put stress in its rightful place. As nursing educator Dr. Roz Seymour said, "Don't focus on stress. You know if you see things as stressful, they will be." Deborah L. Roush, a nursing educator at Valdosta State University in Valdosta, Georgia, advises, "Look at what you can control and what you can't. If you can't control it, move on with a positive outlook and make changes related to what you can control."

Sometimes you will be acutely aware of what's bugging you and whether or not you have control over the situation. For example, if it's late Sunday night and you have a huge test next morning on the entire musculoskeletal system, and all you know for sure so far is that the leg bone connects to the foot bone, you won't need to consult a therapist, a minister, or a psychic to help you realize why you're feeling uneasy.

If you are feeling just overall panicky and anxious for no immediate reason, however, you won't be able to tell if you have control over the situation because you don't know what the situation is. Sometimes journaling can help you in these kinds of cases. Just sit down with a piece of paper (or a whole notebook), start with the heading "I feel upset because . . .," then write until your hand starts to cramp. You may think the problem is the paper that's due next week, but when you finish brainstorming, you may find that you're feeling guilty about not spending enough time with your kids. If you write in your journal regularly, it can help you see patterns in your moods that you might not recognize any other way.

Helping ourselves: the art of self-care

It was no surprise that many of the nursing students I surveyed were hard put to take the time to involve themselves in stress-busting activities like play, meditation, or exercise. As nurses, we are often very good at taking care of other people, but there is certainly room for improvement in how we care for ourselves. There are signs, however, that an effort is being made at some schools to support nurses—and nursing students—in developing healthier behaviors. The RN to BSN program I attended had a required class that included a number of assignments that targeted ways we could improve our own health. This is by no means rare; the University of Minnesota and several other nursing schools have added a "health concepts" course, in which students are required to assess, plan, and reevaluate their own lifestyles (Weisensee, Anderson, and Lapp, 1989).

Maintaining balance

If you've been in nursing school for even a month, you've probably come to realize that you could study 24 hours a day, 7 days a week, and still not learn everything there is to know. Although good study skills and time management are important (and are treated elsewhere in this book), the natural reaction is to simply push harder, which doesn't always move us closer to the goal. Jill Hall, a California nursing student who returned to school after a hiatus of 20 years, tells how she climbed out of this trap: "The worst thing about nursing school stress for me is the constant pressure. During the semester it only increases and never eases. For the first two semesters, I dealt with it by just working harder. Now I take time to play on the Internet and try to walk, swim, or bike every day. I also try to spend more time with my friends."

Jill adds: "When school starts and the novelty value is as high as the workload, it is easier to focus on school alone. But as one progresses at lightning speed through the classes, the social isolation (or is that High Risk for Loneliness?) increases and the need for a life becomes evident. How about treating this nursing diagnosis with an intervention? My suggestion is balance. You need to remain focused on schoolwork, but you also need some relief to keep yourself sane. To new students, I would suggest that you make an appointment once a week to do something nice for yourself. It can be as simple as taking a bubble bath, spending time with your significant other, or going for a long walk."

J.W., a BSN student in Arizona, agrees: "While this might contradict the advice you hear elsewhere, my personal survival tool is not to accept that my personal life has changed too much. My grades are better than average, although not what they could be if I studied more. However, I am sane and healthy."

To what Jill and J.W. suggest, I would add: Take the time to develop a new interest, or renew an old one, about the time that you are starting nursing school. Perhaps you think that taking up skydiving, getting involved with the campaign of a local mayoral candidate, or starting a tattoo club will only add to your stress. But if you pick your activities carefully, you may find yourself invigorated by the change of pace.

I've found that having something that you do well and enjoy doing helps keep your self-esteem intact when the rigors of nursing school threaten to destroy it altogether. For example, my second semester into my AD program, I began to write a semimonthly humor column for a small community paper. There were days when I came home from class and would have preferred to eat my own weight in broken glass rather than sit at my computer and attempt to be funny, but the effort helped me focus on something other than school. In addition, when I look back at the sarcasm in those early columns, I realize I was letting off a lot of steam, too!

The endorphin lift you can get from exercise is also an effective mood elevator and should be seriously considered as a stress-busting technique. Try to pick a fun activity so you'll stay with it. In addition to giving your body a boost, you may find that some of your best problem-solving ideas come when you are swimming, running, biking, or hiking.

When your brain is a pain: recognizing cognitive distortions

Sometimes we can cause stress for ourselves by our negative thoughts. According to the book *Managing Your Mind* (Butler and Hope, 1995), these common negative thoughts are called "cognitive distortions" and can lead to anxiety and depression if not recognized.

The first cognitive distortion is called *catastrophizing*. I call this the "Chicken Little Syndrome." It happens when you have one bad experience and become convinced it's the end of the world. Example: Viola Viscosimeter's study group ran overtime and she is now 7.3 minutes late to pick her kids up from school. Her train of thought, which is on a runaway track and in imminent danger of derailing, goes something like this: "Oh great, the kids are probably standing out in the cold shivering and wondering if their mother even loves them. They are going to feel completely neglected and grow up to be serial murderers, and anyway the authorities are going to take them away from me because I'm such an awful parent, and then the board of nursing will never give me a license. I'll still have all my loans from school, but I'll lose my job because they heard I got turned down for a nursing license, and I'll end up broke and penniless and alone, living on the street."

Another cognitive distortion is *all-or-nothing thinking*. This happens when a person evaluates their performance or personal qualities based on extreme, all good/all bad categories. Example: Peter Paronchyosis's patient in Bed A is ringing for some pain medication and Peter can't find the nurse who has the keys to the narcotics box. Meanwhile, his somewhat confused patient in Bed B is attempting to disassemble the traction apparatus keeping a broken femur in place. Down the hall another patient, whom Peter is covering for another student who went to lunch, has a dozen relatives visiting and they have just decided that the hallway would a good place to resurrect a generations-old family dispute concerning a lost lawn ornament. Peter's instructor approaches him holding the overbed chart of the patient in Bed A, points to the empty space where the 8 AM vital signs should have been filled in, and says, "Hello, have we decided we don't need to do documentation today?" During the whole bus ride home, Peter doesn't remember how well he handled the chaos of the day and can only think, "I'm too disorganized to be a nurse. I'll never make it."

Overgeneralization happens when a person arbitrarily assumes that a single negative event will happen over and over again. Example: It's Melissa Meson's turn to do a return demonstration on vital signs. She gets picked to have her skills evaluated by a crusty older nursing instructor the students have nicknamed PFOF (for Personal Friend of Flo [Florence Nightingale]). She fails because the PFOF says she let the mercury down at

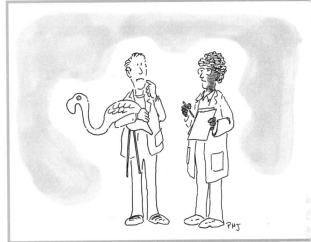

a rate of 1.7 mm per second instead of 2 mm per second. As she leaves the building, she throws her stethoscope into the nearest trash bin, muttering "I might as well quit now while I'm ahead. I'll just get that old bat for next return demo and flunk again."

Selective negative focus happens when a person picks out the negative details in any situation and dwells on them exclusively, which leads them to conclude that the whole situation is negative. For example: Maura Malcontent has moved to a different area of her state because the nursing school there has a reputation as the best in the region. She is used to big-city life and the school is in a rural area. She spends her entire first semester complaining about the remote location of the school ("I'm afraid I'll get mauled by a bear on my way to the dorm! They call this a movie theater? Where are the ATMs around here, anyway?") This causes stress not only for herself but for everyone around her, too.

Disqualifying the positive occurs when a person is confronted with information that clearly contradicts the person's negative self-image or pessimistic attitudes, and the person discounts the information or the source of the information. For example: Dorothy Diamide is convinced that she can't communicate well with her patients in clinical.

At the end of one clinical day, her instructor, Mr. Frankel, says, "You did really well explaining the nonpharmacologic interventions for constipation to your patient today. She was drinking water all morning and asked to go for a walk this afternoon." Instead of enjoying the compliment, Dorothy thinks, "Oh, that stupid ol' Mr. Frankel. He doesn't know anything. Bet they didn't even have constipation back when he was in school."

In the cognitive distortion of *mind reading*, a person assumes that other folks are thinking something and becomes so convinced of the others' thoughts that they don't even bother to check out these supposed perceptions. For example, there was a question on the exam about a subject Brenda Butyric presented to her study group. She is certain that all the members of the group must have gotten the question wrong because she didn't present the subject well enough. Brenda is so sure that everyone is mad at her that she runs from the room whenever she sees anyone from the study group approaching.

Emotional reasoning happens when a person takes the existence of a certain emotional state as evidence of fact. For example: Patrick Pachypodous is sitting in the lecture hall, calmly waiting for the faculty member to pass out the tests. When he receives his, he sees how long it is and begins to panic. His heart starts beating faster, his hands start to sweat so copiously he's afraid he won't be able to hold his pencil, and he suddenly feels like all the knowledge has been sucked out of his brain by a large purple fact-hungry alien. Terror-ridden, he thinks, "I feel like I'm going to fail . . . I must be going to fail!"

You can head these cognitive distortions off at the pass by being aware of their existence and recognizing whether there are certain ones that tend to affect you most frequently. Because it's hard to recognize when your thoughts are causing you stress, you should share this list with a classmate or friend and agree to look out for signs that the other person is the victim of a stress-causing cognitive distortion.

Helping you/hurting me

Understanding codependence

Unless you've been living under a large rock or on the moon, you've probably heard the term "codependent." Originally recognized in people who were in primary relationships with someone who is chemically addicted, it has become a rather vague term, a type of generic insult ("Oh, you're so codependent, whaddya expect?") to be used when you're too old to say "Well, phooey on you."

The phenomena of codependency itself are, unfortunately, still very alive and well. In the book *I'm Dying to Take Care of You: Nurses and Codependence,* Snow and Willard (1990) define professional codependence as "any act or behavior that shames and does not support the value, vulnerability, interdependence, level of maturity and accountability/spirituality of a nurse, colleague or patient" (p. 3). Examples of this type of behavior might include repressing feelings, obsessing, controlling, acting in denial, using indirect communication, caretaking rather than "taking care," and neglecting one's own needs (see *"Caretaking" behaviors*). If you've ever found yourself involved in any of these behaviors, you're not alone. In fact, Snow

---

"Caretaking" Behaviors

Caretaking, a characteristic of codependent behavior, is marked by actions such as the following:

- Doing something we really don't want to do
- Saying "yes" when we mean "no"
- Doing something for someone although that person is capable of and should be doing it for him- or herself
- Meeting people's needs without being asked and before we've agreed to do so
- Doing more than a fair share of work after our help is requested
- Consistently giving more than we receive in a particular situation
- Fixing people's feelings
- Doing people's thinking for them
- Speaking for another person
- Suffering people's consequences for them
- Putting more interest and activity into a joint effort than the other person does
- Not asking for what we want, need, and desire

Source: From *Codependent No More* by Melody Beattie. Copyright 1987, 1992 by Hazelden Foundation. Reprinted by permission of Hazelden Foundation, Carter City, MN.

and Willard (1990) state that "codependence creates harmful consequences for better than 80 percent of the nursing profession" (p. 3).

Although the specific causes of codependence are in dispute, the
generally accepted theory is that codependence is simply a set of behaviors that children learn while growing up in dysfunctional families. I would add that the 0.000001 percent of people raised in
nondysfunctional families can also quickly be conditioned into codependent behavior by situations that encourage indirect communication and situations that require unquestioning allegiance to the idea
that others' needs always come before one's own. Sound like any
hospital floors your know?

It's not particularly surprising that nurses (and nursing students)
sometimes behave in ways that could be labeled "codependent." Often we become nurses because we want to help people, and since
there is a lot more need for help in the world than we could ever individually provide, we can get overwhelmed with trying to meet that
need. In the words of Snow and Willard (1990): "Caring about the
welfare of others is the foundation of nursing as a spiritual discipline. Nursing is also a physical, social, biological and behavioral sci-

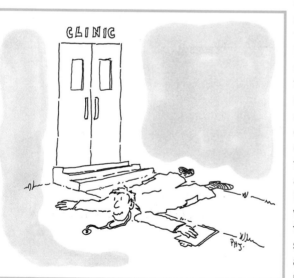

ence. Blending the theoretical and practical ideas from
these disciplines into nursing practice that promotes
care of self in proportion to
the care given to others is
an art. Codependence
draws us off balance into
caring for others at our
own expense, creating professional disillusionment
and personal pain" (p. 3).
In other words, as nurses
we are supposed to care
for others and care for ourselves. When we forget
about the "for ourselves"
part, it hurts us all.

Establishing boundaries

One of the surest ways to rein in our codependent behavior is to
establish good boundaries. "Boundaries" is a term used to mean

limits, particularly limits on what we are or aren't willing to do for other people and ways in which we feel comfortable interacting with others.

During my nun days I had a crash course in the nature of codependence and the consequences of failing to maintain good boundaries. I belonged to a very traditional order, and part of the rule of "charity" was that if another sister asked you for a favor, you were always supposed to say "yes," no matter what the situation. It didn't matter if you were in the middle of sleeping, having a conversation, taking a bath, finding the cure for cancer, or whatever. It didn't take me long to realize that I needed to get out of that particular order because, far from making me a kinder, gentler person, saying "yes" when I meant "no" made me bitter, angry, and very hard to live with. I realized that if you can set—and stick to—limits on what you will and won't do, you will ultimately end up a nicer person than if you don't set any boundaries at all.

Good boundaries are like a "Policy and Procedures" book for our lives that can help things run more smoothly if it's consulted in time. For example, during my first year of nursing school I really struggled with requests from other students to borrow my lecture notes. One student in particular (whom I considered a friend) would skip lectures and then ask to copy my notes 3 days before the test. Not only was this annoying because it meant she didn't have to come to class, but I would always have to track her down to get my notes back. After a whole semester of this, I realized it was making me angry and affecting our relationship. At that point, I had to consider whether I was willing to continue to let her borrow my notes. In the end, I told her that I was comfortable with her borrowing notes from two or three lectures per semester if she borrowed them only at a break during a lecture, went to the library and photocopied them, and brought them back before the end of the break. Setting this limit wasn't easy. In fact, it was uncomfortable because I worried that I would look selfish to my friend. It's possible that she did think I was being selfish. However, after the initial shock wore off, we resumed our relationship, which continues to this day—something that probably wouldn't have happened if I had kept lending her my notes and swallowing my resentment.

In school, you may have to update your "Policy and Procedures" book (your boundaries) on a semester-by-semester or month-by-month basis as new situations arise in the classroom, on the clinical floor, or at home.

Visualization and affirmations

Visualization is the art of vividly imagining the specifics of how we want things to happen—a dress rehearsal for success, so to speak. It is an extremely effective technique for stress reduction because the reaction of your body to a detailed visual picture is pretty much the same as to an actual event. We use negative visualization all the time. For example, pretend you are lying in bed awake before the night of a big test and these are the thoughts going through your mind:

"I haven't studied enough. It's not fair. I could have studied all night and it wouldn't be enough. The material is too hard. I'm not smart enough. Miss Dobkin (insert name of your own most despised junior high school teacher here) was right. I'm just plain ol' dumb. In fact, I don't deserve to take up a space on this planet. I should just quit nursing school and take up raising yaks somewhere in the Himalayas. I'm going to go into the classroom and sit down and forget every-thing I've studied. I'll be so nervous my hands will be shaking too badly to hold the pencil and besides I'll probably throw up on the instructor."

I don't know about you, but I get a stomachache just reading that para-graph! Compare that with the next scenario, in which you are lying on that same bed on that same night, but this time you are thinking:

"I can just imagine what it's going to be like when I take that test to-morrow. I've studied hard, so I know I can do well. When they hand out the papers, I will sit holding my pencil loosely in my hands until I get mine. When we are given the signal to turn over the test, I'll read through the whole thing quickly to get an idea of what it's like. Then I'll start answering the questions, taking care to fill in the little dots correctly! I'll work quickly and carefully, and if I come to any questions that are particularly difficult, I'll remind myself that I've studied hard and that if I just relax the answer may come to me. When I get done with the test, I'll double-check that I've answered all the questions."

I started using visualization when I did my clinical on a labor and de-livery floor. Our group was doing our rotation over a period of time that ended only 1 week before the entire floor was scheduled to be closed due to hospital cutbacks. The nurses, many of whom had worked together for years, were stressed by the prospect of being both separated from a unit and a specialty they liked and being im-minently jobless. There was a lot going on, and nursing students bumbling about and asking, "Uh . . . could you tell me where the Chux are?" definitely didn't help the situation any. To complicate matters further, the nurses used many abbreviations and a lot of nursing slang, and they talked very quickly in report. I sometimes felt too anxious to ask the primary nurse to clarify what was meant, and so I often had to ask later. But after I started spending 10 minutes each "clinical eve" visualizing getting and giving reports, I couldn't believe the difference it made for me. I had the confidence to ask the primary nurse to repeat or explain the things that I couldn't understand, and because my anxiety level was lower, I was able to concentrate better and catch more of what was being said.

Affirmations are very similar to visualization. Affirmations are concise statements of belief that you repeat to replace negative self-talk with positive self-talk (for example, "I am an intelligent, capable student" or "I do well on tests"). They are kind of like yellow sticky notes for your brain, to help you remember what you know is true.

There are lots of different ways to use affirmations. I like to print them up on three-by-five cards and read them (to myself, of course!) when I am on public transportation. You can also use them before you go to sleep or hide them with your drug cards and pull them out at clinical when you need a 30-second self-esteem boost.

Try these additional tips for using affirmations:

- **Keep it positive.** "I am a caring, capable student nurse" works much better than "I will not screw up at clinical today."

- **Keep it simple.** Don't try to run through a deck of affirmation cards big enough to play poker with at one sitting. Concentrate on a few key areas that you need to talk positively to yourself about.

- **Keep it short.** Try "I set healthy boundaries with my family" instead of "I tell my son 'no' when he begs and whines and pleads for something we can't afford at the grocery store." Part of the beauty of this affirmation business is that the affirmations get inside your head, stay there, and pop up when you need them most. Long affirmations just don't pop up as well as short ones.

- **Keep it up.** You might feel funny saying these kinds of things to yourself at first. It may take a little while before the positive thoughts begin to take hold.

No nurse is an island: getting help from others

" a student speaks

"I found that my classmates are my number-one supporters, followed by my spouse. Family/friends had no clue what it was like. Many of my prior friendships don't seem to have survived, but time will tell. Basically, you have to distance yourself from any negative influences, and with your family you just have to be assertive and let them know that when this thing is over you will have more of a normal life. When you're feeling down, I think you'll find that your classmates are your biggest source of support."

— **Jenny Smith, AD, new graduate**

Building your support system of family and friends

Wouldn't it be nice to breeze through nursing school on nothing but brains, raw courage, and double espressos? However, just as it takes a village to raise a child, it takes a big supporting cast to put together a successful nursing student performance.

Assembling your support system can seem more daunting and messy than the prospect of trying to build an elephant out of sawdust, but it's absolutely vital, and the earlier you start, the better your chances of getting what you need. As soon as you make the decision to begin school, start taking stock of your possible supports. By this time, you will probably have talked with most of the important people in your life about this decision and will know how they feel about it. Although it might sound a bit anal retentive, it might be helpful to write each of these folks' names on a 3-by-5 card and put each person into a category such as "positive," "negative," "neutral," or "need more information." On each card you can note any special considerations or limitations that the individual may have—a spouse, for example, might want to be supportive but be working 60-hour weeks and not be able to be much help around the house. Also note any special reasons you want that person's support.

The next step is to get out your trusty planning calendar and phone book and start making calls. Invite everyone who has a card out for coffee (decaf for you, since you'll be drinking a lot of caffeinated beverages in the next few years!) and let them know that your agenda is to talk about your upcoming school plans.

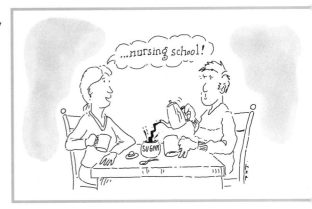

The folks in the "highly positive" category probably will need only a big "thank you" and some specific instructions about how you would like them to support you. If you can, schedule them first because talking to them will give you courage to talk to the folks who are not exactly doing triple somersaults at the thought of your going to school.

For the folks in the "neutral" and "negative" categories, explain that you wanted to meet with them to let them know your reasons for going to school and why it's important for you to have their support. This may be difficult, especially if the person is very close to you (like a parent, spouse, or child) or very set against your decision. Make sure you couch your conversation in as nonjudgmental terms as possible and use "I" statements ("I feel that I need . . ."). Be specific about what you are requesting. "I would like you to take over the responsibility for doing the housecleaning every other week" will help the person understand better than "I really want for you to be on board with me about this."

You may not be able to get everyone to commit to being supportive, but meeting with them in this way starts the dialogue so that the lines of communication are open. Although someone might not change their mind in the 20 minutes that they spend with you that day, it doesn't mean they won't be feel differently 6 months or a year down the road. My partner was originally skeptical about my return to school and especially about my decision to be a nurse. The stress of school contributed to the premature demise of our relationship, but we have stayed good friends and my ex-partner is now one of the strongest supporters of my new career!

a student speaks

"I was halfway through my semester when I realized I was crying practically all the time. Everyone and everything was bugging me; if it wasn't my clinical instructor it was my dog or the kids or our loud next-door neighbors. I tried to just pull myself up by the bootstraps but I felt like the bootstraps kept breaking! Finally, I asked a second-year student if she knew if there was any place on campus I could go for help. I started seeing a therapist at the student counseling center, and it has helped a lot. Every day is still a struggle, but at least I feel like I have a handle on my feelings now."

— J.M., AD student, California

If you need more help

Sometimes the support of your family, friends, and fellow students just isn't enough. In addition to the stress that comes with having the hectic schedule of a nursing student, our work at clinical sites can bring up old issues we thought we had resolved. For example, taking care of very sick or dying patients may bring back grief from a time when we lost someone who was close to us.

profile

"the greatest gift we can give to our patients is ourselves."

Debbie Simone Huff's long career in nursing started in 1969, when she graduated from St. Mary's School of Practical Nursing. She worked for more than 25 years in the ED, CCU, and ICU and says she "got tired of training all the new RNs who were making 5 more dollars an hour than me." So she started back to school to get her RN. In 6 years she was not only a registered nurse but also had an MSN and was a certified clinical nursing specialist in adult psychiatric nursing with a subspecialty in geriatric psychiatry. "I had to start back in English 101," explains Huff. "My kids, and the fact that I loved to learn, helped a lot."

Huff was shocked by how much nursing had changed. "I had been working in small neighborhood hospitals, and when I first went back to school what they were teaching made no sense to me. I realized I had to answer test questions from the point of view of what was in the book, not what I had learned in real life. But I got over my struggle and worked toward my goal because I knew what it was that I wanted."

Huff was interested in integrative medicine and knew that "as a nurse people would trust me more and I would be able to answer more of their general health questions." Huff learned a great deal about herself during her master's program: "I was in some ways an 'old-school' nurse, and in the olden days you didn't move or breathe without asking a doctor. I saw a transition in myself as I went from being someone who takes orders to being someone who gives them."

In 1997, Huff graduated from the University of Pennsylvania with an MSN. She then began to do consulting work for an elder-care company. "The company owned 300 nursing homes on the East Coast, and it was my responsibility to travel to different nursing homes teaching them how to implement programs for people with dementia," Huff says. "I learned a lot about corporate America, and I developed my ability to make decisions and go with them. The job was really a blessing because it afforded me a chance to take classes in integrative medicine. Then the company's stock dropped 40 percent, and that was it for me, but that was a blessing, too, because I was able to apply myself more to other methods of healing."

Huff began her own practice using integrative medicine modalities such as Reiki, hypnosis, and therapeutic touch. Many of her clients are themselves nurses seeking to decrease stress and increase joy in their lives, Huff says. "Learning these integrative methods helps us learn about ourselves. They help us to be centered so we can know who we are and what our strengths and weaknesses are. We need this information so we can take better care of our patients and ourselves. After all, the greatest gift we can give to our patients is ourselves."

Recently Huff was hired by a private mental health organization to implement a program that will provide mental health services for older adults in city-run health centers. She continues to see patients in her integrative medicine practice. "All my practice is very rewarding for me. It fills my spirit. For me, this is the essence of nursing."

When this happens, we may need to expand the circle of our support network to include mental health professionals who can provide individual help and counseling. If you find yourself feeling tired even after a good night's sleep, jumpy, constantly nervous, unable to sleep, or continually sad, or if you have any other emotional symptom that limits how well you can function, you may well benefit from at least an initial assessment.

Seeking this kind of help does not mean that you are sick or weak, and it most certainly does not mean that you aren't fit to be a nurse. Seeking help means just the opposite—that you are strong enough to know what your limitations are and smart enough to know what to do about it! Many people seek therapy because they want to make their adjustment to a new situation as positive as possible. The stress of nursing school is actually an opportunity for personal growth, and a good therapist can help you make the best of it.

Sometimes stress can be severe and we can begin to feel hopeless. If this is the case for you, and if you are having more than fleeting thoughts of hurting yourself or someone else, go as quickly as possible to the nearest mental health emergency assessment center or hospital emergency room. If possible, ask a close friend or family member to accompany you there to help answer questions and provide support.

If you decide that you do want to seek counseling, most schools offer some type of student counseling service; this can be a good option if your health insurance doesn't cover mental health or you can't afford the co-pays, which under most HMO plans run about $25 a session. Usually the services provided through university counseling centers are free, and since these centers are most often on campus, you will probably find their location convenient.

If you have insurance that has good coverage of mental health care (or if you are independently wealthy), you can also seek help off campus. There are a number of ways that you can find a good therapist: You can ask a trusted friend for a referral, call the mental health information hotline that is associated with your insurance plan, or take your chances and pick a name from the Yellow Pages.

Especially if you are picking a name from the Yellow Pages, interview the therapist as though you are considering them for a job—because, of course, you are. Start by asking them their credentials. In some states, anyone with any degree (or no training at all) can set up as a "counselor" or even (in a few states) a "therapist." Also ask what kind of therapeutic modalities they are trained in—for example, some practitioners may specialize in art, drama, or movement therapy. Finally, trust your instincts. The whole point is to feel comfortable enough with the therapist to share how you're feeling; if you don't trust the person, keep looking.

A note about motivation

No stress-busting technique will work if you don't bust your tail doing the work you need to do to be prepared for classes and clinical. Whatever you can do to stay positive and motivated about your school experience will help you feel less stressed overall.

For example, the day I registered for my first nursing school class, I wrote down the seven top reasons why I was going to school. I photocopied them about 3000 times and stuck them up everywhere: in my textbooks, on my walls, even on my alarm clock. (They helped me avoid hitting the snooze button more times than I can count.) I hammered up a miniature version in my closet, where I could see them when I went to get my uniform out. I even had them taped to random cans of soda in the refrigerator. One of my apartment-mates said I was overdoing it when I laminated them and put them up in the shower. My second apartment-mate agreed when she started having dreams that she was studying to be a nurse.

I will probably be finding pieces of paper entitled "Top Seven Reasons Why I Am in Nursing School" strewn around my apartment and among my belongings until I retire, but the motivation they provided was worth it. Craig Moore, a nursing student from New Zealand, said he has a similar system for keeping his spirits and his motivation level high: "Once you graduate here you get a medal (literally). It's a five-pointed star and shows that you are an RN (and that nursing history is militarized). I've got a picture of one in the front of my diary, so that whenever I open it, I see it."

For some other students' ideas for staying motivated, see *Short and sweet motivational tips from fellow students.*

Short and Sweet Motivational Tips from Fellow Students

- Black out every passing day on a calendar and tell yourself, "I can do this."
- Ask a friend who is already an RN to let you see a copy of their license. Picture your name on it and keep that picture in your mind.
- Keep your school bill on a bulletin board over your desk. Whenever you're tempted to skip class or not study, you'll be reminded that you're paying a lot of hard-earned money for your education.
- Go in your closet away from everyone else and practice signing "Your name, RN" on a piece of scrap paper.
- Make up a song about how smart you are. Sing it to yourself.

REFERENCES CITED

Beattie, Melody (1996). *Codependent No More: How To Stop Controlling Others and Start Caring for Yourself.* Minneapolis, MN: Hazelden Information Education.

Butler, Gillian, and Hope, Tony (1995). *Managing Your Mind.* New York: Oxford University Press.

Snow, Candace, and Willard, Dave (1990). *I'm Dying to Take Care of You: Nurses and Codependence: Breaking the Cycle.* New York: Professional Counselor Books.

Weisensee, M, Anderson, J.M., and Lapp, C.A. (1989). "Implementation of a self health project by baccalaureate students." *Nursing Forum* 24: 3–8.

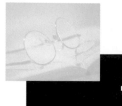

RESOURCES

Books

If you know what you want from life and have a plan for getting it, you will be a much less stressed person in the long run. If you're struggling in this area, I suggest the following titles:

Cameron, Julia (1992). *The Artist's Way: A Course in Discovering and Recovering Your Creative Self.* New York: G.P. Putnam's Sons.

This is the classic on artistic expression and getting beyond blocks to what you really want to do with your life. Suggested daily exercises and a list of helpful resources are included. An integral part of the Artist's Way program is completing daily "morning pages," which involves a specific, stream-of-consciousness journaling technique that I recommend for its de-stressing effects.

Chenevert, Melodie (1995). *Stat: Special Technique in Assertiveness Training.* St. Louis: Mosby-Yearbook.

This is an excellent primer on assertive communication. Chenevert blends together theory with practical tips and even better stories. My favorite is about the nurse who worked in a hospital that once sent the police to her house to ask if she would work on her day off. If you want to know more, you'll have to read the book!

Phillips, Jan (1997). *Marry Your Muse: Making a Lasting Commitment to Your Creativity.* Wheaton, IL: Theosophical Publishing House.

Similar in some ways to *The Artist's Way*, this book also includes beautiful photographs and copious quotes as well as a bit of a social justice underpinning.

Web sites

CODEPENDENTS ANONYMOUS

http://www.codependents.org/

If you recognized yourself in any of the codependency discussion in this chapter and would like to learn more about
breaking free from codependent behavior, consult this site. It contains
information about codependency and links to local Codependents
Anonymous meetings.

THE STRESS DOC

http://www.stressdoc.com/

This is a very comprehensive site about the nature of stress, how to
deal with it, and daily coping strategies. Most of the content is written by Mark Gorkin, LICSW, who calls himself "The Stress Doc. " In
addition to many informative articles, this site also contains the site
author's personal story of how he successfully sought help for mental health challenges.

THE STRESS MASTER SITE

http://www.psychwww.com/mtsite/smpage.html

This is a quick-loading, no-graphics cornucopia of stress-management
information. It details mental techniques for reducing short-term
stress and provides tips for keeping a stress diary, making your work
environment less stressful, and much more.

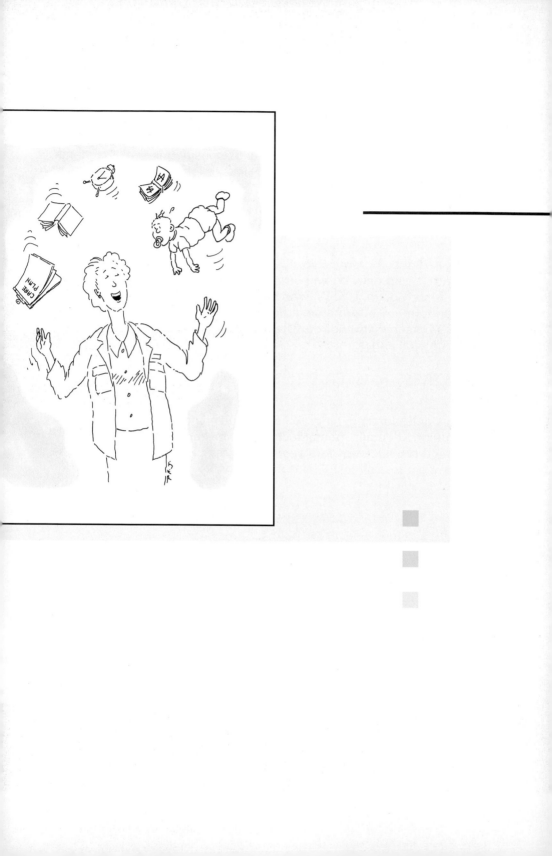

CHAPTER 3

Yes, You Can Avoid: Role Confusion Related to Juggling Multiple Tasks

" a student speaks

"Since I've gotten really busy with nursing school, I've found that I have no short-term memory at all! So I use those little sticky notes to keep track of all the little things and papers I have sitting around. I write things like 'Borrowed Anatomy notes—need to photocopy and return,' or 'Journal article to be used for Nursing History paper.' It's gotten so bad, my husband tells me he's afraid he's going to wake up one morning with a sticky note on his forehead that says 'Husband—sometimes helps with child care and can be used for emergency cooking.'"

— K.M., BSN student, New Mexico

Juggling family and home responsibilities

We've all had those moments. It's the first day of a new semester and you're feeling excited about the idea of learning, of becoming a nurse, and of making a fresh start. You glide happily to class, humming all the way, and find your seat. The instructor starts handing out the course syllabus, and all humming stops when you notice that it looks like an only slightly abridged version of *War and Peace*. Then you open it up and see the amount of work the class requires. Your spirits fall quicker than Wile E. Coyote going down into his cartoon canyon. "Hello," you think, "Okay, I think I can do all these papers and projects and take these tests. But with the 3 minutes I have left over in my day, how am I going to keep my children out of reform school? If I manage to keep them off the streets and keep up with my schoolwork, is my only reward a passing grade, or do I get a Nobel Prize, too?"

Perhaps the most debilitating illness student nurses can develop is what one BSN student calls "MG," or "Mommy guilt": the strain experienced when family and school compete for time. The antidote for this illness is not complicated, but it is rather difficult. In the words of Diane Langton, a family nurse practitioner student in New York, "The key to time management is knowing what you can leave undone and what definitely must be done." She adds, "I waited until my children were in high school, so I had no day care to worry about, but still you have to expect your house to be less clean and be flexible with things like errands, shopping, and so forth. Encourage (ha ha ha) your family to help you."

More information about how to deal with the challenges of being a student while raising a family can be found in Chapter 6. However, some time-management tips mentioned by student-nurse moms and dads I talked to are included below.

Sell the program

Sometimes it seems, as nursing student Mandi Fields joked, that "student nurses don't have a life anymore. Our families and such forget us, and at the holidays we get strange looks because no one even remembers who we are." Even if your spouse and kids want to be supportive, they may be struggling if they feel like they never get any time with you. So, one tip is to remind family members (continually, if need be!) that the changes in your family life are temporary, while the benefits of your going to school will be long-lasting for the whole family. Kids, especially, need to know in concrete terms what going to school will mean for your future and theirs. Talk about increased salary, greater satisfaction with your work, the cool uniforms, whatever it is that motivates you to keep going.

Involve the kids

Other students suggested using creative delegation techniques to help keep you and your family happy. "Think of a million ways your kids can help out," suggested a BSN student from Oklahoma who is raising six kids as a single parent, "and make sure your kids are convinced it's a privilege!"

In my AD graduating class, I had a friend who declared every Sunday night a "Sticking Together Time" at her house. The whole family would make plans to be home for that period, and they would start the evening by ordering out for pizza. Later, my friend's preteen kids would take turns quizzing her from her school notes, and then my friend would help the children with any

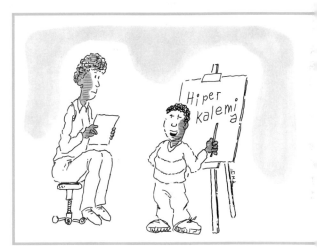

schoolwork they had. While this was going on, her first-grader would be going through the Sunday paper, using his snub-nosed scissors to clip any coupons he spotted, an activity that developed his hand-eye coordination and kept him busy while everyone studied, as well as occasionally saving the family a few cents off peanut butter!

Bundle activities and purchases

Another often maligned but effective technique for maintaining full family and school schedules is "multitasking." I'm not suggesting that you combine activities like shaving your legs and ironing next week's uniforms or cooking dinner and defleaing the dog. But there are daily activities that can be safely and efficiently combined. For example, taking a single kid with you when you run errands can turn a trip to the Laundromat into a chance to catch up with what's happening on the child's soccer team. Listening to lecture tapes while you commute blocks out all the sound of strangers' chatter on the subway and helps you catch up in anatomy.

Another student suggested never buying a single one of anything (except clothes for rapidly growing children). He didn't mean that you should buy an extra car to keep in your driveway in case you might someday need it (although it would be nice to be able to do that, wouldn't it?). He was talking about things like breakfast cereal, bananas, and buttons, which always seem to run out just when you need them the most. In a similar vein, other students suggested cooking a week's worth of meals on Sunday and freezing them. Then, when it's Wednesday afternoon and you're running late after clinical, you'll be able to feed the kids before they start gnawing on your stethoscope in hunger and frustration.

Finally, get extra help if you need it. Pat Reilly, RN, a Pennsylvania nurse who will graduate soon with her MBA in health-care administration, recalled, "The first thing I did when I went back for my BSN in 1998 was to get a cleaning lady. I no longer have the same one, but I refused to give that up when I was finished. I also forced my husband to cook 2 days a week, and I have refused to allow him to give that up either."

Juggling free time and recreation

Many of the students who were quoted in the preceding chapter on stress management mentioned the importance of maintaining balance. That's not shocking—I think one of the hardest time-management tricks is learning when to work and when to play. "It's really easy to spend too much time partying in your first year and procrastinating about all your schoolwork," said Victoria Hunter, a nursing student from Ontario, Canada. "But I found that if I used my spare time between classes to rewrite notes, finish my readings, and such, then I had extra recreational time at night and on weekends to relax. It was hard to walk away from my friends who were talking, eating, and so forth, but it was worth it when I had my weekends free."

Jodi Hancock, a BSN student in Washington State, has a strategy that works for her: "I only do the assignments that are necessary; the extra time is for me." But besides having a generalized work-to-fun ratio planned Into your day, a fundamental question to ask yourself is "What is the best use of my time right now . . . at this moment?" "Right at this moment" is an important part of the question, because sometimes at that moment you may be tired, annoyed, or distracted. If you're on the clinical floor, perhaps you need a quick bathroom break and sip of water. If you've been on a study marathon and there is no possible way you can cram one more fact into your brain, maybe you need to rent a silly movie and call it a night. Although we'd all like to be superhuman, there are some occasions when the very best use of our time is to tumble into bed and take a short (or very long) nap.

Sometimes, however, we don't need a rest, but we need a change. In these situations, I highly recommend spending some time doing community service. Just make sure your choice of volunteer work is very different from whatever is going on at school at the time. For example, if you're struggling through a grueling clinical rotation on an oncology floor, you will hardly find volunteering for a local hospice invigorating. But if you're up to your bellybutton in prerequisites and feel like you're never going to see an actual patient, then spending time at the hospice might be helpful both for you and for the people you encounter. Even if you're very busy, it's often possible to work volunteering into your schedule. As Jessica Wheeler, a BSN student from Connecticut said, "I volunteer for an elderly woman once a week for 2 hours and I find this very enjoyable. I have formed a great relationship with her, and she appreciates my coming out to help her a lot. I think volunteering for community service is wonderful, even if you only have an hour or two a week."

The nuts and bolts of time management

" a student speaks

"I hated—absolutely hated—the unit we had on dermatology in Nursing III. I got grossed out just looking at the pictures in the text! Plus, all the information seemed the same to me, and I never could keep papule, macule, or whatever, straight. I hated derm so much I put off studying for that test until the night before. I passed that unit but barely. If I would have had to take the whole class over because I procrastinated about studying one unit, I would have been really mad at myself!"
— **D.W., BSN student, Georgia**

Dealing with clutter

I decided to include the topics of "clutter" and "procrastination" together because they are such good buddies: Usually one is not found without the other lurking around somewhere. A good example is the very long semester when I took a Statistics class. The class, which is required for graduation from the BSN program, started with the basic assumption that students remember what they learned in high school math. This may be true for other students, but it was most definitely not the case for me, at least partly because I'd finished high school more than a decade before I started that Statistics class. I was somewhat muddled by the first lecture, and by the second lecture I was so confused that all I could do was raise my hand and say, "Ah . . . I don't get it." The more confused I got, the more I put off studying. By the third lecture, all I could do was stare blankly at the instructor while he covered the chalkboard with alien-looking symbols and figures. When it seemed appropriate, I would blink.

I only made it through Statistics with the help of a friend who's a very conscientious student herself, and who knew I was also. She suggested we spend some time studying together for the first test, so we met for lunch one day. As we pulled out our sandwiches and study materials, she gasped. We both looked down at the notebook I had been using for the class. It was crammed full of random papers that were sticking out in all different directions, many of them torn or dirty from being shoved into my backpack. The cover was hanging on by an inch of raggedy spiral wire, and when I opened the notebook, all manner of debris fell out. My friend scratched her head and looked at me with a mixture of concern and bewilderment. "Ah, Kelli . . ." she began. "Didn't you use to be a good student?" I had, up to that semester, been a fairly decent student, and that's exactly my point: Confusion, procrastination, and clutter can contribute to a cycle that leads to failure, even for students who normally do well.

When I was taking Statistics, I kept every piece of paper from class (even though I couldn't summon the energy to arrange them in some kind of reasonable fashion) because I felt out of control, and holding onto all the paperwork I generated made me feel like I was doing something about how far behind I was in class. In fact, I was doing something; but I wasn't doing anything useful. I was only creating clutter, which made the situation seem even more hopeless.

There is really only one remedy for clutter, and that is to be ruthless about tossing unneeded items, especially papers. If you think there is a good chance you might use your high school zoology notes again, it might be worthwhile to keep them, but, as a rule, anything we keep because it "might" be useful someday in the very far off future will end up making our lives more 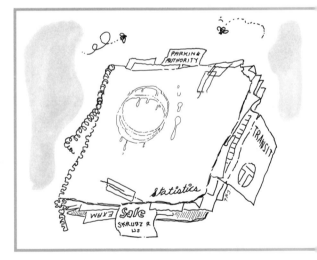 difficult. The fact is that if you keep too many papers sitting around, you won't be able to find the paperwork you actually need.

The second clutter-elimination rule is some wisdom you probably heard first from your grandmother. "If you want to keep things tidy," she would say, shaking her finger at you in her intense but affectionate manner, "don't put things down, put them *away.*" There's much truth in that statement. We all know it's easier to spend 23 seconds putting your lovely, new, sparkling white nurse's shoes away then to spend 30 minutes looking for them the next week, only to find them rapidly being reduced to a mushy white protoplasmic mess by your hyperactive Doberman puppy. It's just so easy to sigh, "I'll do it later" when you come home from a long day.

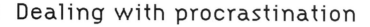

Dealing with procrastination

This conveniently brings us to the subject of procrastination. I have never encountered anyone who doesn't procrastinate, at least to some extent. I once met someone at a party who told me he worked for a small company that required its employees to meet every morning at 9 in front of a large clock in the main office. Facing the clock, the employees would shout "Do it now!" 15 times in unison before starting their workday. He said this exercise helped boost productivity. I said it sounded like a cult, which kind of ended our conversation right there. But, irrespective of a few overzealous professional motivators out there, most of us underestimate the toll that procrastination takes on us.

Many of us put off doing our taxes, a great deal of us put off regular vehicle maintenance, and nearly everyone I know puts off going to the dentist. Procrastination in these areas wastes time and can be detrimental to our financial state, our cars, our teeth, and our self-esteem. But procrastinating with schoolwork is an especially difficult problem because our educational system breaks each learning module into very short segments, usually semesters of 16 weeks. This leaves little time before procrastination causes very big problems. By procrastinating, we put ourselves in a situation where it is impossible even to say that we gave it out best try.

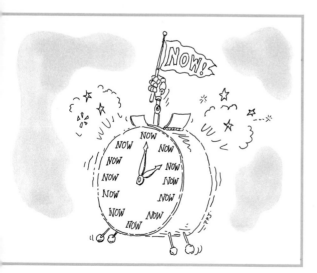

If you're going to make any progress against the procrastination habit, it helps if you can figure out exactly why you're procrastinating. For example, in the case of my Statistics course debacle, I put off studying because I found the material difficult. Of course, this made no logical sense, since unless aliens abducted me and switched my brain with that of someone more mathematically inclined, I was going to struggle with statistics no matter when I studied. And because I left a great deal of work to do until the end of the semester, I was under a lot of pressure to figure things out quickly. This certainly didn't help my information retention.

Another common reason for procrastination is fear. This most often comes into play when we are afraid we're going to fail at something. For example, let's say Nancy Nursingstudent has a very generous-minded instructor who gives her 3 whole weeks to write her first care plan. She's heard the instructor has fairly high expectations for care plans and she feels overwhelmed by the task, so she ignores the assignment for the first week. The second week comes and she sits down at her desk to work, but suddenly the *Leave It to Beaver* marathon that her dorm-mate is watching on TV seems absolutely fascinating. The third week comes and she is in bed until Wednesday with some kind of nasty flu. When she starts to feel better on Thursday, she gets a little panicky about the impending deadline, so she goes to the library to really buckle down for an evening. Once she gets to the library, though, she is dismayed to find that she doesn't have all the information she needs from the patient's chart. Now desperate because time has almost run out, she drives full-speed to the hospital, pulls into the area marked "Loading Zone Only," screeching on two wheels and nearly wiping out a handful of innocent bystanders waiting for the bus. She double-parks and runs up the 15 flights of stairs to her clinical unit (the elevator is broken, of course). Searching for the patient's chart, she finds that the patient has been discharged and that the chart was sent down to medical records 7 minutes before she got there. A crestfallen Nancy Nursingstudent does what she can and turns in a very vague care plan on Friday morning. She isn't surprised when she gets her care plan back with a big "C minus—barely passing" scrawled across the top in red felt-tip pen. "Hummphh," she grumbles, "I never thought I could do a care plan anyway." She didn't think she could do the care plan. That was exactly the problem!

Once you can get a handle on why you're procrastinating—whether it's the obtuse material or your gut-wrenching fear or whatever—you can deal with the problem directly. However, that isn't always enough to make sure we stay on task and focused. This is where you can make peer pressure work for you. Dr. Rosalee Seymour, a nursing educator from East Tennessee State University, suggests a simple but effective intervention: "At the beginning of every semester, examine requirements for each course you're taking and put all due dates in your calendar. Then mark at least 2 weeks before each due date as *your* due date to take the work to a peer for review."

Working while in school

" a student speaks

"I worked in an assisted living facility as a nurse's aide the last summer before I started my clinicals, and I think it was a great experience. I was ahead of most everyone because I had seen and done stuff they hadn't. I had witnessed two deaths and learned postmortem care. I knew how to do ADLs and how to ambulate and transfer. It was a great experience, and I think you should get some kind of experience in the health field during your academic career, especially if you have any doubts. I don't know if it will help me get a job after graduation, but I'm sure it will look great on a resume."

— Jessica Wheeler, BSN student, Connecticut

If you can afford not to work

The vast majority of nursing educators I talked to, while understanding of students' need to work while in school, were less than enthusiastic about combining full-time studies with anything more than part-time employment. Nursing educator Judy Reishtein, of Wilkes University in Wilkes-Barre, Pennsylvania, had this advice: "I recommend that students cut their school year employment to the absolute minimum their budgets can afford. Nursing requires many hours of study and clinical preparation, and students who work full time (and overtime) do not get the full benefit out of clinicals or classroom instruction. More time spent studying during the school year can save many hours of grief later on (for instance, if they flunk state boards)."

Some students were also adamant about the damage that can happen when work and school compete for time. One student, who had an older sister who flunked out of nursing school because she tried to combine classes with a 40-hour-a-week job, said, "I'm not going to make the same mistake my sister did. This is too important to me. I am willing to consider taking out loans, borrowing from my parents, selling magazines door to door, or starting a lemonade stand to avoid neglecting school by working too many hours at my job."

Another option—perhaps more practical for traditional-age students who are less likely to have the financial responsibility for dependent children—is to look for a job that has the flexibility to accommodate your fluctuating schedule. Nursing student Victoria Hunter said, "I had a part time job around 15 or 20 hours a week from my second to my fourth year. I wouldn't recommend it to a first-year student, but once you have a good idea of how much time your schoolwork will consume, then you can judge how much time you have for a job. It helps if your boss is flexible, too. Working on campus can also make your schedule easier."

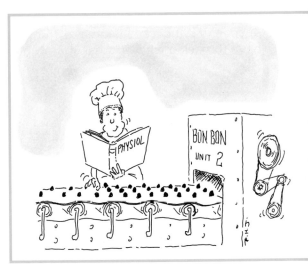

Getting (or keeping) a job in health care

For many students working is not an option, but a prerequisite for survival. "[Working while in school] often accompanies the need to eat, as well as to feed our children," said MSN student Sandra Wolf. "I am reminded of Maslow's hierarchy. Isn't food and stuff at the bottom?"

For these students, a job in a health-care setting can provide income and learning opportunities. "Working [in a health-care environment] is definitely helpful if you use it as a clinical experience. File those experiences in the back of your brain as you work," said Diane Langton, a family nurse practitioner student in New York State. Jenny Smith, a new AD graduate from Oregon, adds, "The best jobs are working on call in a hospital or in a nursing home. Usually they are willing to work with your schedule, since they are the most understanding of your career goals."

Still, it is smart to evaluate your ratio of work to school time frequently in order to make changes as needed. "I think work is an individual thing," said Deborah L. Roush, a nursing educator at Valdosta State University. "Work can support learning, but only if the mind is alert enough to process what is to be learned. I do not judge the work situation but ask students to look at what stressors they can reduce, and if the issue is time to study versus time to work, then they have to decide what is most important to them."

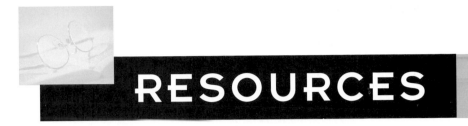

RESOURCES

Information in your mailbox

Many good Web sites provide free e-mail newsletter subscriptions, offering you a good way to keep up with clinical information without having to search the Web or skim nursing journals on your own. Here are two:

KAPLAN CENTERS

www.kaptest.com

You can read about the NCLEX here, as well as sign up for a free e-mail service that will shuttle study tips to your mailbox at the rate of around two a week.

MEDSCAPE

www.medscape.com

Register free to search the database and sign up for their e-mail service, which will send summaries of new research articles to your account once a week.

Web-based time-management tools

I highly recommend Web-based planners for coordinating schedules. There are a number of Web-based calendars and most have the same basic features, so your best bet is to log on to a few and see which one suits you. Some of the most poplar web-based planners are the following:

COMPASSNET WEB ORGANIZER

www.compassnet.org

This site has a very easy-to-use and cute format (you have to give them your annual income in British pounds before they'll let you register, but don't worry—they don't check up on you!). The site has a calendar, address book with a "click to send e-mail" option, and a very easy-to-use bookmark file with the option of putting the bookmarks into easily labeled subdirectories.

DAYTRACKER ON LINE
www.daytracker.com

This site looks very cool as it downloads; it contains a very large calendar area and allows you the option of setting up threaded discussions and bookmarks. It even allows you to track your stock portfolios, which you might have lost sight of in your haste to memorize the cranial nerves for that big exam.

FAMILY NET
www.familytime.net

This site has free software they will send at your request that includes a family calendar, menu planner, areas for recipes, a coupon organizer, and home record storage. It's good for the busy student trying to run a household, probably less so for a traditional-age student living in the dorm.

ONELIST COMMUNITIES
www.egroups.com

Onelist is especially useful for study groups. You can create your own e-mail list, maintain a shared calendar that you can set up for all the members, and keep an optional archive of all the postings. You can also keep shared files, such as lecture notes for that killer Anatomy and Physiology exam coming up next week.

SUPERCALENDAR
www.supercalendar.com

This site might be the best option for families because it allows you to combine four or five calendars into one for easy reference for all involved. It is also very pretty to look at. Supposedly its graphics-intensive environment provides "activity at a glance" functions, but it might be visually distracting for some people.

YAHOO PLANNER
www.yahoo.com

This is perhaps the simplest and quickest-loading of the free Web calendar offerings. It provides you with e-mail, a file manager, a to-do list, and a place for managing files.

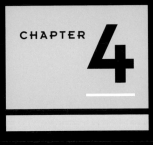

CHAPTER **4**

Yes, You Can Avoid: Impaired Memory Related to Information Overload

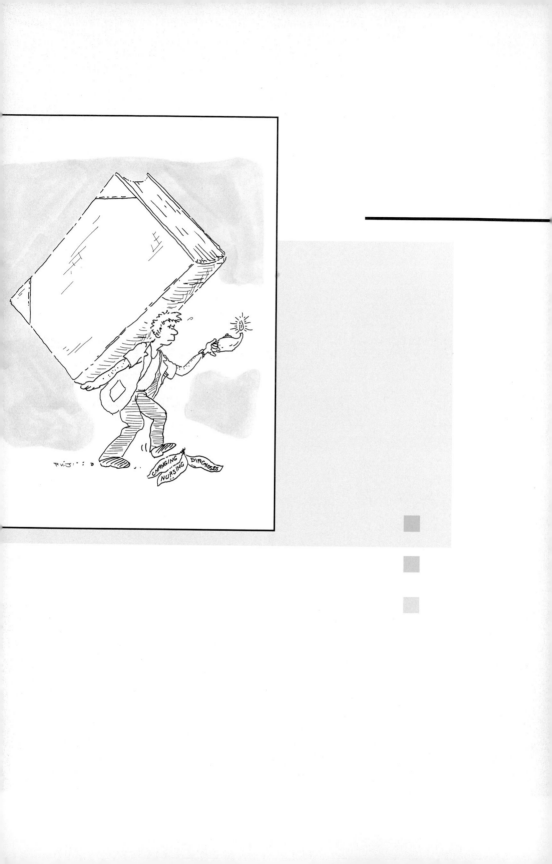

CHAPTER **4**

Yes, You Can Avoid: Impaired Memory Related to Information Overload

a student speaks

> "I thought I was a good student. Then I went to nursing school. I found out that the frantic reading and the studying I did before a test in my other classes was what I have had to do every single doggone day in Concepts of Nursing I. I needed all the help I could get just to stay afloat!"
>
> — S.L., BSN graduate, Florida

Congratulations! You've chosen a nursing program and school, gotten in, figured out how to pay your bills, and set up a time- and stress-management plan. The fun just keeps coming; now you have to do the actual work of being a student nurse. It's perfectly reasonable to panic at this point. You may even feel like locking yourself in the bathroom to cry and exclaim "What have I done!" over and over until your toddler breaks down the door and demands a peanut-butter-and-jelly sandwich.

Such fear, while certainly understandable, is not warranted. If you have even a modicum of confidence in your school's admissions process, you can remind yourself that the school has probably decided you can actually do the work required of you. Besides, if you've gotten this far, you must already have some redeeming study habits, which, with some fine-tuning and a lot of effort, can get you through nursing school without a gray-matter meltdown. In this chapter you will learn some effective tips and techniques for sharpening your classroom and study skills as well as how to apply your existing skills in the unique environment of nursing school.

Finding a guide

As you begin, I highly recommend making friends with someone who is a year ahead of you in school. Besides supplying moral support and living proof that, yes, someone has survived this process before you, your second-year friend can give you all sorts of tips about what to expect and how to study. Some schools provide mentoring programs, pairing first-year students with second-year students for this very purpose. If this is the case in your school, your mentor may or may not actively seek you out. It's up to you, then, to seek out your mentor.

If your school lacks a mentoring program, you may need to be clever about meeting someone who's willing to be your nursing school pal. Why not try bribery? For example, if you know where on campus the second-year students go to study, you can have pizza sent to them before a big exam. You can ask if they need any photocopies made, or volunteer to iron their uniforms. You can even stand just outside their clinical site with a bottle of white shoe polish and offer to give their shoes a quick touch-up as they rush in to get report. All this rather transparent groveling may irritate some folks, but others may be flattered or at the very least take pity on you. Either reaction will achieve your purposes. If you can choose your second-year mentor, try to find someone who is realistic about the nitty-gritty of nursing school but who isn't so burned out that they've become cynical.

Reading: How much is enough?

students speak

"I bought all the required texts (I was a geek and still am), but after buying three different nursing diagnosis books in three semesters because a new one was recommended every year, I learned that recommended books weren't always necessary. Often they would only assign one chapter out of a recommended book, so I would go to the library and copy it. I tried to do all the reading but it was not humanly possible, so I usually gave up mid-semester. It didn't usually help anyway, because I learn better in a lecture than by reading a book."

— Laura Baker, BSN graduate, New York

"I purchased all the required books and I had to. I definitely needed them. I would have failed if I hadn't done the reading, since my professors put stuff on the tests from the books that wasn't in our notes. It also helped to read in the book what we had learned in class because it reinforced everything. It definitely pays off to read."

— Jessica Wheeler, BSN student, Connecticut

When you get the syllabus for your first nursing class, you may be overwhelmed as you page through the list of 7.2 million required and recommended books. The thought of sprinting to the bookstore and plunking down your hard-earned cash (or precious credit card) for books you'll never read even if you live to be 597 years old may even send you back to the bathroom for another full-fledged panic session.

Not surprisingly, many nursing educators I talked with said reading every page of every required and recommended text was imperative to nursing school success. Most students I talked with, however, did not always read all the required texts and seldom got to the titles on the recommended reading list.

So before you bar that bathroom door, take a deep breath and put in a call to your second-year nursing school friend. Ask if you can take them out for a cup of coffee (have you noticed how closely success in nursing school seems to be linked with taking folks out for coffee?) and go over the syllabus together. Although classes will vary somewhat from year to year, particularly if the instructors change, the basic body of knowledge remains fairly constant. Your new confidante may be able to give you a general idea of how much of the material you must know is covered in lecture and how much comes from outside reading.

The idea here is not to "get one over" on the instructors by reading only what you know is going to be on the test, or to coast through nursing school without ever cracking a book. The fact of the matter is that assigned and recommended reading in nursing school is practically unlimited, and distinguishing what you really *need* to know from what you would really *like* to know may make the difference between passing and failing a test. Dr. Rosalee Seymour, a nursing educator at East Tennessee State University, suggests that the best way for students to manage their reading load while in school "is to know that they cannot read it all and learn how to read quickly and select out what is important."

Making the most of your reading time and effort

" a student speaks

"Almost everyone I communicated with started school with the intention of completing each and every reading assignment before each lecture and, without exception, no one has been able to do it! My last 2 years (of a 5-year BSN program) consisted almost exclusively of studying from the study guides and lecture notes from an upperclassman buddy, and rarely did I read the textbooks. The reading was more important during the first 3 years because there was a lot more stuff to be memorized or just read over and over and over in order to get close to understanding concepts (like acid-base balance)."

— Deborah Bower-Mays, BSN graduate, New Jersey

Pre-lecture reading: to read or not to read

Instructors and schools differ in how they encourage students to read before coming to a lecture. Every class day, the instructor for my first-year skills lab gave a 10-question quiz about the assigned reading. The quizzes weren't used as part of the grading process, but a student who scored less than 60 percent on more than three quizzes could be dropped from the program.

We all did our reading.

In this case, our decision was simple: Read before class and pass or don't read and fail. Although this hard-nosed approach to pre-lecture reading seemed a bit excessive to us then, we were grateful at exam time because we already had a good handle on the material covered in skills lab. We could then concentrate on studying the material from the nursing lecture.

If you suffer no immediate consequences from neglecting the pre-lecture reading, it becomes more difficult to find the time and discipline to do it. However, it doesn't take an expert in educational psychology to figure out why instructors assign and encourage pre-lecture reading. Not only does completing pre-lecture reading have the long-term effect of making studying for tests easier, but it also provides a foundation for understanding the lecture.

Instructors (at least the more optimistic ones) prepare for a lecture with the idea that students have some basic knowledge of the subject matter, since this is what the assigned reading is supposed to provide. While on some days you may be able to waltz into lecture having not so much as glanced at the book and find yourself able to follow along quite nicely, you'll never know what you could have absorbed if you had read beforehand. Plus, on some days you may be so confused that you'll feel quite sure the person giving the lecture is actually a mutant alien from a distant planet where they speak a language that has not even the slightest similarity to English. On these days, you will want to ask a question or two, and if you have not done the reading, it will be painfully and embarrassingly obvious.

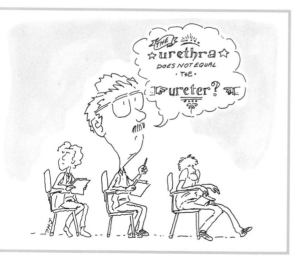

Even if you're not particularly easily embarrassed, those "I-haven't-even-looked-at-the-material-and-so-I-need-the-instructor-to-spoon-feed-me-the-information" questions are guaranteed to make you unpopular with students and faculty alike. Nothing is more annoying to a room full of students trying to understand the intricacies of urinary system physiology than a student who pipes up from the back, "Wait, wait, wait. The urethra and ureter . . . are they the same thing?"

In a perfect world we would all do our assigned reading before the lecture and come to class prepared, notes from the text in hand, bright-eyed and eager to learn about the marvels of our chosen (and revered) profession. However, real life tends to interfere with nursing school, and so sometimes pre-lecture reading gets pushed lower on our list of priorities by the need to communicate with a distressed spouse, strip the yard of poison ivy, or play a game of Parcheesi with a sick child.

If you can't do your reading

There will be days when you won't be able to read before the lecture for some reason. How do you minimize the effect that not reading before lecture has on your grades and, ultimately, on your ability to pass boards and work as a nurse?

First, it helps if you can verbalize why you are choosing not to read any given assignment. This cuts down on rationalizations because you hear how flimsy your excuse sounds. For example, if you say out loud, "I am making a conscious decision not to read for Monday because that old bat Miss Bensen is doing the lecture and I can't stand her," you'll quickly realize how self-defeating this reasoning is. On the other hand, when you say, "I am making the conscious decision not to read for Monday's lecture because I am going to have my gallbladder out tomorrow at 6 AM and need my rest," your choice sounds much more reasonable. That is if, in fact, you are having your gallbladder taken out.

Second, prioritize, prioritize, prioritize. (Are you sick of hearing that word yet? Don't nursing instructors just love that word?) For example, if you are having a hectic week and have time to read only 2 of the 17 chapters you've been assigned, concentrate on chapters containing material that is especially difficult or unfamiliar to you.

Optimizing your reading time

Since the time and energy we have to actually read in nursing school is limited, but the reading is not, it's important to find ways to optimize the reading we do during the time we have.

FIGHT DISTRACTIONS

Although it may seem somewhat self-evident, maintaining concentration is one key to increasing reading effectiveness. Time spent looking at words and turning pages is not equal to time spent comprehending. It helps to minimize distractions in the environment, but unless you have a study area buried in an underground cave or secluded in a virgin wilderness, there are always going to be some stimuli vying for your attention. Even if you can somehow eliminate external distractions, we are all capable of producing all sorts of internal distractions that can be just as annoying.

One method students have used to learn to ignore distractions involves placing a check mark on a conveniently located piece of paper each time they find they aren't concentrating. Some people find this helps them become more aware of the amount of time they spend daydreaming and redirects them back to the task at hand. There are two advantages to this system; one is that it can be used to document your reaction to both external and internal distractions, and the second is that it can provide ongoing documentation of your ability to concentrate (or not) at different times and places. You can use this information to fine-tune your reading and studying system because it helps you choose times and places to study that work best for you. I sometimes use this technique, but I occasionally find that the act of making a check mark on the page actually reinforces how distracted I am since I have to momentarily remove my eyes from the text to deal with making the mark.

A variation of this technique is useful when you have 8 trillion things on your mind and 8 million pages to read. When you find yourself distracted by problems or things you're worried about getting done, write down the problem or task and place a check mark beside it if you find yourself worrying about it instead of concentrating on the task at hand. I've found this to be extremely helpful at times. Perhaps the act of writing down the task/worry/problem assures our "inner worrier" that we will deal with it when we have time.

BOOST COMPREHENSION

There is more than one way to increase your reading comprehension, and perhaps by now you have one that works for you. The most basic thing you can do to enhance reading comprehension is to have a clear idea of why you are reading. When you sit down to read, ask yourself (although probably not out loud, unless you're in that soundproofed cave we talked about earlier), "What is the point of me spending my time to read this material?" For example, are you trying to memorize facts? Understand a complicated physiological process? Obtain a working knowledge of an issue?

Then, as you read, stop after every main topic, paragraph—or sentence if you have to—and ask yourself, "What did I just read? What does it mean? Why is it important? How does it apply?" If you are reading clinical material and have started your rotations, try to relate the information to someone for whom you have provided care. For example, you won't forget the physical changes that sometimes occur with longtime steroid use if you've ever seen a patient with a so-called moon face.

Another way to reinforce what you've read is to take notes or outline as you go. If your instructors have a tendency to put questions on the exam that come directly from the book (rather than testing solely on lecture content), these notes may come in handy when the time comes to study for an exam. However, if you find that your instructors don't usually ask questions about topics from the book that they didn't cover in lecture, extensive note taking may just slow down your reading without yielding much real benefit.

Many students underline in their books as they read, whereas others think underlining is a complete waste of time. Although underlining may not increase comprehension and retention the way that taking notes does, it may help you interact with the text and move from passive to active reading. Underlining also provides a handy way to pick out important points when you go back later to study the reading in a more in-depth way. Sometimes, though, I go back to what I've underlined and think, "Good grief! Why did I think that was important?" It's a good idea to underline in pencil so you can erase the marks

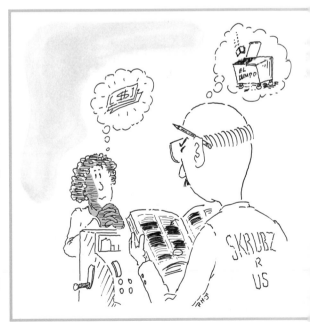

if you find you've been off track. This has the additional advantage of greatly increasing the chance that the bookstore will be willing to buy back your used text if you find yourself strapped for cash when you go to buy books for next semester.

SPEED YOUR READING

Some students are satisfied with their reading comprehension but are frustrated with the amount of time it takes them to read assignments. A few nurse-educators I talked with suggested taking a speed-reading course before beginning nursing school. If you have the time and money to take such a course, it will probably be helpful, but it's probably not necessary to weep bitter tears if you can't fit it into your budget and schedule. Often you can increase reading speed simply by paying attention to how fast you're reading and making a conscious effort to read more quickly. It helps if you have an idea of how fast you usually read a specific type of material. For example, it's doubtful you will be able to read your pathophysiology text as quickly as you read Nancy Drew mysteries as a teenager. Use this information to keep track of improvements in your speed. Obviously, if your comprehension starts decreasing as your reading speed increases, you'll have to slow down a bit, but you'll probably still be reading faster than before.

Learning from lecture

Attendance, preparation, and general classroom behavior

If you are thinking about cutting classes tomorrow, you might want to think again. You have paid for your instruction (or someone else has). If you don't go to class, you are paying a rather large sum of money to teach yourself. The nature of classes is that they build on one another, and if you miss one class, it's that much easier to miss the next one, and the next one, and the next . . . well, you get the picture.

Also, going to class gives you that little boost you need to stay interested in the material. Remember when you only kept up with *The*

Old Man and the Sea in high school because you wanted to know what folks were talking about in class? The same principle applies here: Attending class can keep you interested in the material, since even the most boring lecture will pique your curiosity at some point.

Of course, you've probably heard the standard advice to sit near the front of the room during lecture. This is certainly a good idea if your attention tends to drift when you sit in back or if you have trouble seeing the chalkboard or other visual aids if you're seated more than 5 feet away from them. However, I talked with a number of good students who said they prefer to sit in the middle rows or even in the back of the room. Why? Well, some instructors like to do the spontaneous questioning thing ("So, Larry, tell us what you know from the reading about intracranial pressure measurement . . ."), and they often target students sitting up front because they have the most eye contact with them. If you get nervous because you're afraid you might be questioned, you may find that you have a harder time concentrating when you sit in front. Also, if you have trouble sitting still, or are nursing a nagging cough, your classmates will appreciate your not sitting front and center and distracting them from the lecture.

If you aren't going to sit in front and you are in a good-sized lecture hall, make sure you do at least one thing every day to ensure that the instructor notices that you are in class. No, I'm not suggesting that you throw spitballs or bring a basket of unshelled walnuts to class and crack them open as soon as the lights go down for the slide show. Instead, ask a well-thought-out question at some point during the lecture. (For tips on asking intelligent questions, see *The art of asking a good question*.)

If you don't have a question to ask, walk by the instructor on your way in or out of class or on a break and give them a big smile. Call it kissing up if you will, but this action serves a vital function. First, if you have a problem or get behind and need to go to the instructor for extra help, they are going to be a lot more eager to help you if they know that you have been doing your part by coming to class. Second, this small gesture can help you maintain a positive attitude toward the instructor. It's easy to demonize an instructor, especially if you are really struggling in a particular class. It definitely won't help your days go any more smoothly if one instructor starts representing all that is bad in nursing school, your life, and the world in general. Three seconds of human contact between the two of you can help decrease these negative feelings and allow you to concentrate on the work at hand.

The Art of Asking a Good Question

DO . . .

- Ask an instructor questions based on his or her experience (for example, "Is what you're describing a common clinical occurrence?")

- Formulate your question carefully and make it succinct, especially in large lectures.

- Speak for yourself, not the whole class.

- Ask the question in question form.

- Be persistent about getting your question answered, even if you are meeting with resistance from students or instructors who are trying to rush the lecture along.

DON'T . . .

- Bother asking, "Is this going to be on the final?" Apparently, every educator since the beginning of time has heard these eight little words ad nauseum. Sometimes, however, it isn't clear whether the material presented is just "FYI," or introductory matter, or an amusing anecdote, or whatever. In those cases, it's appropriate to ask the "Is this . . ." question, but word it differently.

- Jump ahead and ask questions about the parts of the handout that haven't been covered yet.

- Be afraid to ask questions that seem basic—for example, the definition of a word or acronym.

- Ask questions of classmates. It's distracting to other students and the instructor.

- Ask questions that can be found on the syllabus.

- Hesitate to ask questions that piggyback on another student's questions, but DON'T put down another student's question with your own.

I'm sure I don't need to mention how helpful it is to come prepared to class. Reading the material is a large part of this preparation, but having all the equipment you need makes life easier, too. I became quite infamous in my Anatomy lecture for never showing up with a pen. Both my classmates and I were relieved when I started packing my bookbag the night before the lecture so that I would actually notice my lack of a writing instrument and take corrective action. In addition, packing the night before gives a small psychological edge. Having my bag packed and things in order always makes me feel like

I'm going on a special field trip in pursuit of wisdom, instead of just showing up for another lecture on gastroesophageal reflux disease.

A note about notes

Everyone has their own individual way of taking notes in class that works for them. A common method (and one detailed by many guides to college studying) is to divide each sheet of note-taking paper down and the middle and write the key points of the lecture on the left side of the paper and add the details on the right side. This makes the information easy to review, although I've found that it

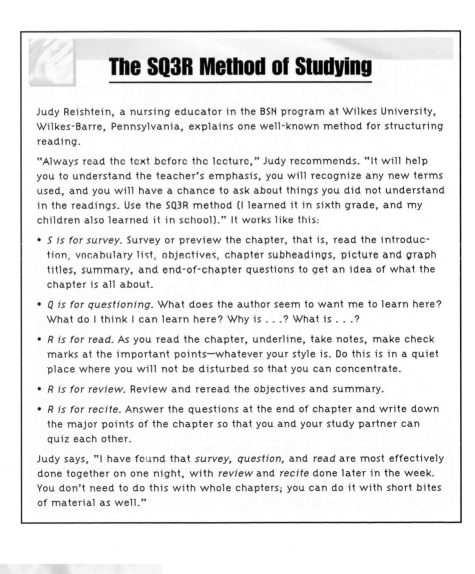

The SQ3R Method of Studying

Judy Reishtein, a nursing educator in the BSN program at Wilkes University, Wilkes-Barre, Pennsylvania, explains one well-known method for structuring reading.

"Always read the text before the lecture," Judy recommends. "It will help you to understand the teacher's emphasis, you will recognize any new terms used, and you will have a chance to ask about things you did not understand in the readings. Use the SQ3R method (I learned it in sixth grade, and my children also learned it in school)." It works like this:

- *S is for survey.* Survey or preview the chapter, that is, read the introduction, vocabulary list, objectives, chapter subheadings, picture and graph titles, summary, and end-of-chapter questions to get an idea of what the chapter is all about.

- *Q is for questioning.* What does the author seem to want me to learn here? What do I think I can learn here? Why is . . .? What is . . .?

- *R is for read.* As you read the chapter, underline, take notes, make check marks at the important points—whatever your style is. Do this is in a quiet place where you will not be disturbed so that you can concentrate.

- *R is for review.* Review and reread the objectives and summary.

- *R is for recite.* Answer the questions at the end of chapter and write down the major points of the chapter so that you and your study partner can quiz each other.

Judy says, "I have found that *survey, question,* and *read* are most effectively done together on one night, with *review* and *recite* done later in the week. You don't need to do this with whole chapters; you can do it with short bites of material as well."

uses up a great deal of paper. For another common and well-respected studying structure tool, see *The SQ3R method of studying.*

If you have trouble keeping up with the lecture, try taping the class. This can leave you free to concentrate more on understanding without having to take meticulous notes, since you can always go back and fill in the gaps later when you listen to the tape. Several students told me they used this method successfully. Some also mentioned that they later used the tapes to study while running, doing the laundry, or driving to school.

Finally, always try to review your notes shortly after class so that you won't be stuck 15 weeks down the line trying to figure out what "P.L. = DP- LM ^^^^ " means. Reviewing right after class allows you to clarify with other students what you don't understand. Remember, however, that the instructor is the one who makes up the test questions and (most likely) is the person with whom you will need to plead if you contest a test question. So when in real doubt, seek the instructor out.

Planning your study time

Efficient use of study time and effort is often a result of choosing a location that works best for you. Many traditional students favor the library as their study location of choice, away from the dorms and the noise and temptation of pizza parties, phone-booth-stuffing contests, or loquacious roommates.

If the library is not close to where you live, or has limited hours, you may find it helpful to find a public place where you can study undisturbed. The park is ideal in nice weather, as is a public library or a friend's house (especially if no one is home). Another viable option is one of those oh-so-comfortable chain bookstores/cafes where you can have a latte while you practice with your Littman (stethoscope) or write a care plan for a post-op transurethral resection patient while drinking tea. The advantages of any of these places is they get you out of your home/dorm/apartment, where distractions (including a bed that can look mighty inviting no matter how long it's been since you've changed the sheets) abound.

Some students told me they became very superstitious or obsessive about their studying location. I prefer the term "steadfast." For example, during my first semester I found a place in the 24-hour study room at my school that was not too hot or too cold, nor too bright or too dark. It wasn't so close to the entrance door that I was interrupted every few seconds, or so far away that I felt like I was running a marathon every time I had to get up and go to the bathroom. It was also next to a picture window that had a great sunrise view. In order to get that certain spot on a weekend, I would have to be there by 7:00 AM.

Once I got to My Special Study Spot (doesn't that sound like an educational TV show for kids?), I would guard it jealously, growling at any med student who dared to cross my path. This choice of location served two purposes. First, it reminded me that I was sitting at My Spot for one purpose only: to study. Why else would I leave my apartment, walk 10 blocks, and brave the cold or snow or heat or wind or whatever the environment was putting out that day at such an early hour? Second, always studying in one place gave me an edge when test time rolled around. Sometimes when I was in the midst of taking a test and was stumped by a question about something I knew I had studied, I could go back and imagine that I was in My Special Study Spot. The memory of being in My Special Study Spot ("Oh, yeah, I remember, it was a Saturday morning and I was drinking orange juice and scarfing down a green eggs and ham sandwich. The sun had just come up and . . .") would trigger the memory of the fact or concept I had learned.

When you have a ton of studying and reading to do, remember the old adage, "It's easy to eat an elephant, if you do it one step at a time." (Although I daresay that the person responsible for this adage most likely never actually ate an elephant or they wouldn't be nearly so glib about it). If you have three books to read, a care plan to write, and several thousand note cards to memorize, break each activity 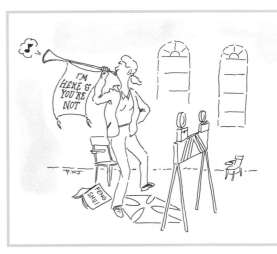 into tasks that are small enough that you can actually imagine getting them done. Also, since concentration usually falters after about 50 minutes of intense work, try building a 10-minute break into every hour of studying. For more ideas about how you can use even the smallest bits of time for learning, see *Studying on the go.*

Studying on the Go

Here are some time-saving tips suggested to me by busy students:

- "Put all the material you need to know on 3 × 5 index cards. This makes your studying instantly portable."

- "A good way to keep up with all those note cards, which can add up quickly, is to punch a hole in one corner and run a key-chain ring through them. You can get almost 150 cards on a small ring. Put them in your purse or backpack. Pull them out wherever you are. You will be amazed about how adding 5 minutes here and there helps. This takes a little bit of multi-tasking ability. But with the cards on the ring, you don't have to worry about dropping the bottom 20 when you are going over the one that has you stumped. I try to get all the cards for the chapters that are on the next test on one ring."

- "Write particularly difficult concepts on heavier-weight paper (tag board, for example) and laminate it. Then you can study in any number of places that would normally be too humid, such as the shower, the bath, and so forth."

- "If you have social events you feel obligated to attend but you really can't afford the time out from studying, make what you are trying to learn the subject of conversation. I went to a party once and talked about nothing but cranial nerves the whole time. People actually seemed interested, but perhaps they were just being polite. However, this approach might tend to decrease your social invitations over the long run."

- "Don't worry so much about your books getting messed up. I study every day while I eat lunch and my original med-surg book was so stained and gross my wife made me keep it in a closed plastic bag when it was on the shelf. She says it will probably attract roaches. She may be right, but I have a 4.0 in my nursing classes!"

- "Practice your assessment skills with seldom-seen relatives at your family reunions. They won't say 'no' since it will give them a rare chance to interact with you, and you won't be embarrassed because you see them so infrequently."

Joining a study group

" a student speaks

"An advantage of a study group is that it is not healthy to drink alone! Laughing at/with and helping one another is helpful and satisfying. Misery does love company. If you understand a concept enough to explain it to a friend, you can get it right on a test and it's good to share how you learned it, too."

— Sandra Wolf, MSN student, Wisconsin

Pros and cons of study groups

Both nurse-educators and students had mixed views on the use of study groups while in nursing school. Ann B. Fives, a nurse-educator from Raritan Valley Community College in New Jersey, listed some advantages: "[With a study group] students can see things from different perspectives, and work can be divided into smaller segments, with each student researching one aspect of a problem or assignment and then sharing. Also, commitment to the group keeps students on a studying schedule." She also notes some disadvantages: "A slower student may slow the group down, or a persuasive student may convince the group that their perspective is right, and conflicts can arise."

Some students cite lack of time and large geographic distances between students as reasons for not joining a study group. At least one student I talked with found the entire idea of study groups quite ludicrous. "We [students] spend all day, every day with each other. I mean, I see my classmates at 6:45 AM on clinical days before our coffee has had a chance to kick in! I like my fellow students, but I would never ever willingly spend extra time with them, even if it meant that I could get a 100 percent on every exam. Enough is enough!"

Choosing groupies

Deciding whom you study with is as important as deciding whether you will participate in a study group at all. Most study group members I talked with agreed that participants should be well matched in terms of motivation so that students can build on each other's strengths. Many students stated that they occasionally felt frustrated when one member of their group continually arrived at study sessions unprepared.

Jessica Wheeler, a BSN student in Connecticut, said, "I think it is good to study with people who have the same study habits as you and do the same on tests. If one person can just read over their notes and know the material, then [studying with them] won't really help you."

Judith Reishtein, a nurse-educator at Wilkes University in Wilkes-Barre, Pennsylvania, concurred with this advice but suggested that there should be some diversity in the group. "At least one person in the study group should be the compulsive type who takes dictation rather than notes (her notes are almost verbatim transcripts of the lectures)," Dr. Reishtein said. "If possible, one should be strong clinically and the other strong in classroom theory. Choose study partners who are strong where you are weak (they can help you learn what you don't understand) and weak where you are strong because you learn best when you try to teach someone else."

Building a structure

a former student speak

"I am a firm believer in group work. Split the reading load and share notes. Each group member needs to take responsibility for the quality of his or her notes. After sharing notes from the readings, use the notes to guide reading and make additional notes as needed. That streamlines the reading and yet gets the job done."

— Deborah L. Rousch, nurse-educator, Valdosta State University, Valdosta, Georgia

A study group can be as informal as a pretest cram session or as structured as a trio of students who meet after each lecture to review the material. The only nonnegotiable point is that everyone must agree on what the group's goals are. For example, when I was working on my associate's degree, I studied with a small group of people the 3 nights before each exam. I used my time with the group to increase my understanding of difficult or complicated concepts. I can sincerely say that I would never have gotten through cardiac phar macology without the group's help. Our group was very informal. In fact, one guy always brought a basketball and bounced it against the wall in an annoying fashion whenever we covered a particularly difficult topic. Despite the fooling around, we were all agreed that no one would show up for study sessions with absolutely no knowledge of the material. Our informality worked for us, but it might have driven a more detail-oriented person to drink (seltzer with a twist of lime only, of course).

One of the biggest benefits I got from my group was that the other members helped me to be realistic about my material. I would come in with 1324 fact-crammed note cards, all stressed out about what I didn't know. Recognizing that I usually overstudied, someone would inevitably grab the cards from my hand and pretend to read (mocking my voice): "On page 345 of a text that we weren't even required to read, what was the caption under Figure 23-A?" Their good-natured teasing gave me some much-needed perspective and helped me realize how much I actually *did* know.

Elizabeth Wheeler, a nurse-educator in both a generic BSN and an MSN program, related this story from her days as a student: "[Our study group] used to allow a certain amount of de-stressing time and then get to the work at hand. Something I remember most vividly from one group I was a part of is when one of us just couldn't seem to understand the positions of the infant's head as it came through the birth canal.

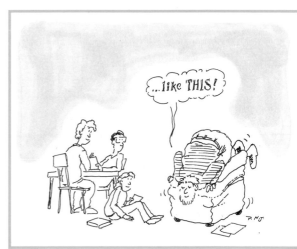

One group member, a kind of portly, bearded guy, took it on himself to explain it to her and the rest of us. To this day, some 20 years later, I have a picture in my mind of him kneeling on a hassock, head down, pretending to be born. None of us will ever forget those positions, to be sure."

This brings me to a final and crucial suggestion about study groups: Make sure everyone in your group has a well-developed sense of humor. Nursing school is too serious for you to avoid spending a great deal of time laughing. For more information on "Humor for Healing," see Appendix B.

A note on competition in nursing school

a student speaks

"I found that everyone in my nursing class is very cooperative and not that competitive. If one person does bad on a test, then we try to help them do better on the next test. We help each other out so that we can all just survive. I don't think that anything in the academic/clinical setup encouraged this. There is some competition in the clinical setting that I've noticed. I think some clinical instructors give special attention to some students. There was competition over who had/has the hardest/easiest patient. Some were extremely jealous if one person got to do a ton of skills in clinical while others didn't.

— Jessica Wheeler, BSN student, Connecticut

When I sent out my original book outline to student reviewers, I said the book would include a short section on dealing with competition in nursing school. The reactions I got were quite extreme. Some students thought competition was a big problem at their school and should be addressed extensively, while others denied it was a problem and urged me to devote page space to something that was, in the words of one reviewer, "more positive." I think it's important to recognize unhealthy competition (the kind that impedes teamwork) in its primeval form before it gets a grip on us and we act as vectors, spreading it to the workplace as graduate nurses. Competition is universal. We all want to feel like we've done well. And who are we going to compare ourselves to besides our peers? But as we compare ourselves, we need to remember that any grade we receive is about how well we did on one particular test or assignment. After all, a grade—or a grade-point average—may be wholly unrelated to our actual ability to perform as a nurse when the time comes.

Obsessing about how your grades compare to those of others can also make you discouraged. If you compare yourself to the class genius who gets 99.99999 percent or better even on the tests that everyone else fails, you could start thinking, "Oh, woe is me, how did I ever get into this? I'm never going to be a nurse, I'm not even fit to be a dogcatcher, I should never have been born . . ." This is both uncomfortable and unproductive. If, however, you compare yourself only with Joe Slouch who has come to class twice since the semester began and once appeared on the clinical floor in a maroon tuxedo, you may be lulled into a false complacency.

Eight Ways to Avoid Unhealthy Competition

- If grades are posted by PIN numbers, keep yours private.
- Don't participate in the "whadyaget" game after test results are posted.
- When you work in a group, make a conscious effort to include less verbal or assertive members and to solicit their feedback.
- At clinical rotations, always be on the lookout for peers who might need a hand for tasks such as turning a patient or making a bed for a patient in traction. Also, accept assistance graciously when you need it.
- Refuse to bad-mouth other students behind their backs.
- If possible, deal with conflict at the source. If you are having problems with a classmate, try to solve it directly with them.
- Use humor judiciously to defuse tension, but be conscious of others' feelings and the fact that stress can make even the hardiest individuals sensitive to good-natured ribbing.
- Actively look for traits and behavior to appreciate in your classmates.

For some helpful information about competition and cooperation, see *Eight ways to avoid unhealthy competition* and the Resources section at the end of this chapter.

Papers and such

" a student speaks

"Why do we have to write papers? I want to be a nurse, not a best-selling author."
— **M.P., AD student, New Jersey**

Researching

It's only a matter of time until you will be confronted with an infamous "lit search" assignment, if you haven't already. A "lit search" simply means looking for what has been written about a certain subject. For example, let's say your instructor assigns everyone in class a research summary paper on any aspect of health promotion they choose. That's a pretty wide-open field, so you choose "Managing cardiovascular risk factors among residents of the North Pole" as your topic. You then use databases (two commonly used in undergrad nursing programs are the Cumulative Index to Nursing and Allied Health Literature [CINAHL] and Medscape) to find what research, if any, has been done on this population. Let's say you don't find anything in your initial search. Does that mean nothing exists? No, because perhaps if you add the search terms "Claus" or "elves" on your next try, you will find that the Centers for Disease Control and Prevention has sponsored several studies relevant to your subject, including ongoing trials of the efficacy of genetically engineered eggnog on cholesterol levels of North Pole residents.

Finding the right combination of search words takes time, patience, and perseverance, and possibly a little bit of help from a reference librarian. When you're doing research, reference librarians are your very best friends. Find out who the reference librarian is at your school and get in good with this person. Offer some home-baked cookies, free car washing, baby-sitting services, whatever it takes. It is the reference librarian's business to know the ins and outs of finding information. They will not only help you find the literature or data you need, but also enable you to find information the next time on your own.

Many allied health databases are now available online, but few have searchable full-text articles available, which means you still have to schlep over to the stacks to pull a journal article and photocopy it. However, the number of peer-reviewed journals that are online only is increasing. While it is certainly important to use good judgment when evaluating online information, there are many good data sources in cyberspace. A few Web sites to get you started are listed in the Resources section of this chapter. Be forewarned, though: Some technophobic instructors refuse to accept any kinds of Internet citations in a formal paper, so make sure you know how yours feel about using these kinds of resources.

Writing strategies

Some students feel like engaging in a primal scream session when anything that resembles a written assignment is thrown their way. However, if you have the time, motivation, and a carefully selected topic, you may find that that you come to enjoy doing research papers. (Do I sound like a parent brandishing cod liver oil?) Here are some suggestions to help make the task easier.

When you get the syllabus and see a written assignment, make absolutely sure you understand what the instructor is asking for. You should have a general idea of what type of assignment it is (literature summary, research paper, etc.) and know the criteria that will be used to grade the paper. It's important to get these questions cleared up sooner rather than later. If you're e-mailing your instructor these questions at 11 PM on the night before the paper is due, they are going to be (rightfully) annoyed and (rightfully or wrongfully) prejudiced against your paper. Of course, it sometimes happens that projects are finished at the last minute. This fact does not, however, need to be advertised to the instructor.

Pick a topic for your paper with great care. Be extraordinarily cautious in choosing to write about any topic on which your instructor has published extensively or is considered a worldwide expert. While the instructor may be delighted that you are interested in their area of expertise, you may feel so pressured to turn in a perfect paper that you risk being overwhelmed by the task. Also, pick a subject based more on your own interests and less on how much information is easily available on the subject. If you are genuinely curious about a subject, ferreting out well-hidden sources of information will be fun.

Additionally, you can streamline your papers and research projects by choosing similar topics for many of your assignments throughout your nursing school career. For example, I am interested in how the concept of harm reduction can be applied in different community health settings. For my Health Promotion class, I completed a research project about needle exchange as a harm-reduction tactic for injection drug users. For my Research and Theory class, I wrote a paper detailing the ways in which different health education theories can be applied to develop programs that might reduce the harm from undertreated hypertension in homeless adults. For my Maternal and Child Health concentration, I developed outreach materials for a nurse-managed health center that used harm reduction as its theoretical basis. My instructors might have been very weary of reading about harm reduction, but I enjoyed every paper/project I did. I also developed a large library of information that I could use for later projects.

Spend the most time on the features of the assignment that count for the most points. For example, when I was writing a paper for a Developmental Psychology class, I was careless with some of my bibliography citations. I had not looked carefully enough at the syllabus to see that each messed-up citation earned a 4-percentage-point deduction. I did fairly well on the content part of the paper, but I got an 81 percent because of the points lost from the references. If I had looked more closely at the guidelines, I would have spent more time double-checking the proper format for references and less time making sure I used "affect" and "effect" properly.

Finally, proofread, proofread, proofread. It is always difficult to go back over your material "just one more time," usually because you're sick of the subject or have become attached to your words and don't want to change them. However, a final proofreading, done if possible by an objective third party, can greatly enhance your paper's readability. Don't depend on your word-processing program to catch all spelling errors and typos. It may flag a gross misspelling of "platypus" but cannot always tell if you typed "he" when you wanted to use "the." Finally, if you can avoid doing the last edit of your paper on the computer screen, you will catch more sentence-level errors. Alternately, you can read the paper backward, which also makes it easier to catch typos.

Don't forget to keep copies of everything you give an instructor, both on hard copy and on disk. This will save much time and heartache should the instructor misplace your work. The stereotypical "absent-minded professor" may be more prevalent in disciplines other than nursing, but there's no sense in taking any chances with your hard work.

RESOURCES

Web sites

CELLS ALIVE
www.cellsalive.com

I would never have thought that anyone could be this excited about bacteriophages. This site is a well-illustrated if somewhat overenthusiastic guide to cells. It's an excellent help if you are struggling with microbiology (don't miss the section on HIV replication!). As an added bonus, when you're done studying, you can investigate its extensive collection of free e-postcards of microscopic entities. Go on—you know you want to send that postcard of the animated dust mite to your hygiene-impaired roommate.

EMERGENCY NURSE CLIP ART COLLECTION
www.emergency-nurse.com/resource/clipart/clipart.htm

This site features adorable pictures of ambulances and syringes as well as anatomical line art and other items you might need to illustrate slide presentations and projects. All are uncopyrighted and free for the taking.

FUTURE NURSES
www.efn.org/~nurses/

Future Nurses is a student-oriented Web site maintained by a recent ADN graduate from Oregon. This site includes study tips, sample tests, dosage-calculation tools, some student nurse humor, the full text of the Nightingale Pledge, and a collection of links to other helpful sites. It also includes an extensive acronym list that may be helpful for those nights when you sit at your desk thinking, "I know there must be another meaning for SOB."

THE INNER BODY
www.innerbody.com

This site somewhat inexplicably compares the inner workings of the human body with the inner workings of a car, which will leave you rather befuddled if car innards are not your hobby. Still, the site's full-color, animated presentations of some basic anatomical processes may be helpful to many students. If you are struggling to learn the path that blood takes through the heart, this is definitely the place to come. It also contains an interesting section on the intersection between human anatomy and human history. Don't you want to know why wealthy women of the late nineteenth and early twentieth centuries needed "fainting couches"?

LOYOLA UNIVERSITY MEDICAL CENTER STRUCTURE OF THE HUMAN BODY PAGE

www.meddean.luc.edu/lumen/MedEd/GrossAnatomy/GA.html

This is an extensive, well-illustrated anatomy site. Don't miss the List of Anatomical Threes and the Bone Box feature.

MEDICAL MATRIX

www.medmatrix.org

This site is a relatively comprehensive portal and search engine for peer-reviewed information on the Web. It requires registration, but registering is free.

NATIONAL LIBRARY OF MEDICINE PUBMED

www.ncbi.nlm.nih.gov/PubMed

This is another search tool for finding scientific literature. You can search for abstracts online and match citations (for example, if you have part of a citation but need to find the rest). There's also a cool clinical query feature that allows you to narrow down searches to literature regarding only prognosis, diagnosis, or treatment of a disease or condition.

NATIONAL LIBRARY OF MEDICINE VISIBLE HUMAN PROJECT

www.nlm.nih.gov/research/visible/visible_human.html

I love it when the U.S. government does something useful! This is the home page of the Visible Human Project, originating at the National Library of Medicine. The project provides extremely detailed images of anatomical structures to help students of all types learn about the human body. Read their fact sheet for more fascinating details and check out the links to different sites that make use of the images.

THE NATIONAL WOMEN'S HEALTH INFORMATION CENTER LIST OF ON-LINE MEDICAL DICTIONARIES AND JOURNALS

www.4women.gov/nwhic/references/dictionary.htm

Hooray for folks who use white backgrounds and make their Web pages easy to read and fast to load. This site contains pages and pages of links to online journals. It's best suited to broad searches when you want to see what kind of general information on a topic is available on the Web.

THE NATURAL PHARMACIST

www.tnp.com/encyclopedia.asp

This is a commercial site with an eye to selling you its products, but if you can ignore the ads, the site provides an excellent encyclopedia of drugs that interact with natural remedies. Because it's completely referenced to mainstream, peer-reviewed journals, you can use the information as a source for even the most persnickety prof's papers.

PROFESSOR FREEDMAN'S MATH HELP PAGES

http://www.mathpower.com/

Professor Freedman is a faculty member at Camden County (New Jersey) Community College, and is she ever enthusiastic about math! This site is full of tips, links, and resources all about college-level math. There's even a special section on math anxiety.

THE TABER'S DICTIONARY ONLINE

www.tabers.com

Taber's is not free; full use of Taber's online will set you back $29.95 a year, but it's definitely worth it. You can look up more than 55,000 vocabulary entries, check out the hyperlinks to cross-references, study the illustrations, and, best of all, listen to an audio of hard-to-pronounce medical terminology. It will save you the embarrassment of mispronouncing "medulla" when speaking with your clinical in-structor. You can also access a more limited version of Taber's for free at The Internet Drug Index, *www.rxlist.com*.

TULANE UNIVERSITY ACID-BASE TUTORIAL

www.tmc.tulane.edu/departments/anesthesiology/acid/acid.html

This tutorial on acid-base balance was developed by the Department of Anesthesiology at Tulane University. Comprehensive and rela-tively easy to use, this site contains more detailed information than you will probably need to know for Anatomy 101. However, if you know all this information, you will definitely pass your acid-base exam!

THE TWELVE DAYS OF ANATOMY

www.homepage.montana.edu/~awmsg/student/twelve.html

This site makes for a great anatomically correct study break. Someone at the University of Montana's medical school definitely didn't have enough to do.

UNIVERSITY OF CHICAGO HEALTH WEB ANATOMY

www.lib.uchicago.edu/hw/anatomy

This is mostly a collection of annotated links to take the guesswork out of finding multimedia and interactive Web tutorial sites for anatomy. It loads quickly and is easy to search.

UNIVERSITY OF PENN INTERACTIVE KNEE

www.rad.upenn.edu/rundle/InteractiveKnee.html

This is a very cool, if somewhat specialized, site that illustrates the human knee and how it works. It starts with basic information and gets progressively more complex.

UNIVERSITY OF WASHINGTON MUSCLE ATLAS

www.scar.rad.washington.edu/muscleatlas

This site allows you to look up the origin and insertion of each muscle. You can search by body region or muscle name. Full-color illustrations and a self-test feature are included.

WASHINGTON UNIVERSITY MEDICAL SCHOOL GUIDED TOUR OF THE VISIBLE HUMAN

www.madsci.org/~lynn/VH/tour.html

This quick-loading and chatty site is possibly the easiest to use of the virtual human Web sites, although the information it contains is somewhat less comprehensive than that in other sites.

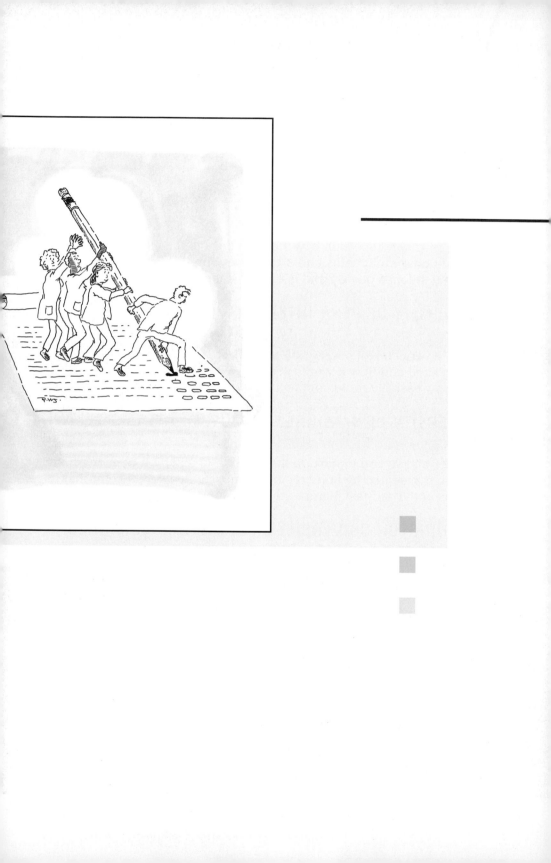

CHAPTER 5

Yes, You Can Avoid: Anxiety Related to a life Built Around Multiple-Choice Tests

" a student speaks

"If I take one more multiple-choice test, I think I may become physically ill. I won't be able to help myself. Can't they think of any other way of assessing how much we know?"

— F.C., AD student, Iowa

Most students I interviewed for this book mentioned that test taking was one of the most stressful events in their journey through nursing school. At least one said that the *"irrationality* of tests" (her words) was her number-one stressor. This is not particularly surprising, since at many schools multiple-choice exams are the only determinants of grades in core nursing classes. How well you do on these tests determines whether you pass or fail the course; what's more, core nursing classes are worth so many credit hours that the tests can greatly affect your grade-point average. In some schools, clinical performance is given a numerical grade that is added to a student's overall GPA, but in many others it's pass/fail. Unfortunately, this prevents demonstrated excellence in the clinical area from helping a student's course grade.

If you let your grade-point average drop below a certain point, you could be put on academic probation, lose your financial aid and your self-respect, cause the stock market to career wildly out of control, and reverse the force of gravity. Well, realistically, you could end up on academic probation and lose your financial aid.

Many nursing schools use multiple-choice tests as their sole grade determinant for core classes because they believe studying for multiple-choice tests prepares students for the NCLEX. The thinking behind this is that if someone is competent or even awe-inspiring in the clinical arena but can't pass the NCLEX, they won't be able to work as a nurse anyway, so it would be unfair to allow that student to graduate. A cynic, however, might say that nursing schools try to keep their first-time NCLEX pass rates high by weeding out clinically capable students who struggle with multiple-choice exams and might need more than one try to pass boards. Regardless of which view you hold, there are ways to increase your chances of success with these exams.

Preparing mentally for tests

Playing private detective

Assuming you're reading, going to lecture, and keeping up with the material, the next step in succeeding with exams as they are given at your school is to snoop for all the exam-related information you can obtain. Start with your syllabus. It should include information about the number of exams you will have, the amount each will count toward your grade, and at least a general description of the material each exam will cover. This is important information that provides the structure for the rest of your search.

The syllabus may also include other handy information, such as how many questions will be on each exam and what parts of the material will be emphasized more than other parts. If you can't find this information written anywhere, ask the instructor. If you are shy, ask after class or (like I did) plead with a more verbal classmate to ask for you. If you don't wait until the last class before the exam to ask, chances are excellent that the instructor will not turn into a purple people eater (or any other color people eater for that matter) and yell at you for asking. The instructor will probably be glad someone is thinking ahead.

Another important piece of information to obtain is who writes the exam questions. If only one faculty member gives lectures, you may not need to spend too much time worrying about this. However, you will need this information if the class has been team-taught or if there have been a number of guest speakers.

Finally (and most importantly), study your instructors. Of course, they are doing their best to provide information in an unbiased way and to test over all the material evenly. However, they are human beings (not purple people eaters) and so have their own idiosyncrasies and thoughts about what material is most important. For example, one instructor may quiz endlessly in class about the nursing process; it's a safe bet that at least a few of his exam questions will involve nursing diagnoses.

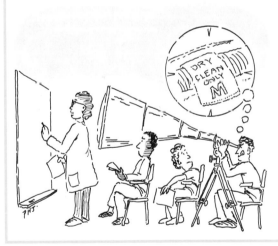

If it's not obvious, ask about your instructor's area of specialization and whether they still practice. An instructor who is clinically current may ask more application questions than one who is not. Try to figure out if they have any special philosophical beliefs. Do they talk about the "good old days," bemoan the loss of the cap, and think nursing students today are "unruly and undisciplined"? This is a red flag that they may write more difficult test questions, and you should perhaps spend more time on the material they covered. In all these situations, you have to use your own best judgment about how to focus your studying, based on what you have come to know about the instructor. Talking with your "buddy" from the year senior to you can also help.

Using practice tests to prepare

" a student speaks

"A second-year student told me about using NCLEX books to prepare for tests. I couldn't believe how much more confident it made me feel. Hello—why didn't someone tell us about this earlier?"
— Tom Amalia, BSN student, Arizona

Like Tom, I was surprised by how much practicing with NCLEX review books helps with preparation for tests while still in school. If you haven't yet done so, run to your closest bookstore and buy one or two comprehensive NCLEX review books. I don't suggest buying these types of books online because they are relatively cheap and massively heavy, so what you end up saving on the cost of the book gets eaten up by shipping and handling costs. Especially helpful are books that have a number of sample questions broken down by content areas. Suggested books are included in Chapter 8. Many of the same publishing companies that put out the NCLEX review books also produce NCLEX review card decks. These can be useful for studying on the go.

You can use the questions from these books to see how instructors may ask about certain topic areas and to practice answering the kinds of questions you could be asked. The questions can also tip you off to content areas you may have missed.

Supplement your practice testing with reviews of the past year's tests, if they are available in the library. Be sure to compare content if the instructor has changed; the material covered may remain essentially the same, but you don't want to lose out if it doesn't. One particularly good way to review with old tests is to use them in study groups to quiz each other. You can even make a big production of the quiz and have it serve double duty as a stress-relieving game. Give

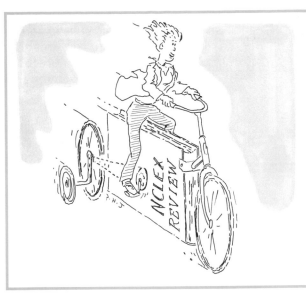

prizes for things like the most correct answers, the most bizarre answer, or the contestant most likely to have a myocardial infarction during the exam.

Part of the goal of exam preparation is to be so well rehearsed that you won't be surprised by anything the instructor throws your way. Note: This "throwing your way" is strictly metaphorical. If anything not metaphorical (e.g., a purple bowling ball, a large striped bass) is thrown your way, I humbly suggest transferring to a different school.

Preparing physically for tests

Rest and exercise

When exam time rolls around, sleeping on a schedule becomes particularly important. Your brain needs beauty sleep, too, and unfortunately, you can't stay awake for days on end, then sleep before the night of the exam and expect your natural brilliance to return.

I'm not saying that you should miss your daughter's wedding or the pregame ceremony in which you are supposed to be crowned homecoming queen so that you can catch that requisite shut-eye. However, it is essential to commit yourself to a routine that includes appropriate amounts of nightly sleep.

Of course, it helps if the important people in your life support your sleep schedule, too. Your realistic commitment to sleep 7 hours a night will be in vain if your roommate thinks that 3 o'clock in the morning is an excellent time to practice the oboe or invite the folks down the hall in for a primal scream therapy session.

In these cases, naps can be lifesavers and, best of all, you can catch them where you can: in the library between classes or while waiting for your order to arrive at a particularly slow restaurant. I have a weekly appointment that takes me out to a remote suburb and, if I have nothing I need to study, I sleep all the way there and all the way back. Note: This works particularly well if one is using public transportation but not well at all if one is driving.

Exercise is a great stress reliever and can help to promote sleep, as long as you don't try to run the Iron-Nurse Marathon in the 30 minutes right before heading off to bed. When I was getting my associate's degree, I established a pretest ritual of going for a short swim. The ritual helped me feel prepared and together, even when I was not. I continued my ritual when I went to take the NCLEX. Unfortunately, the blow dryers at the gym chose that very day to malfunction. I'm sure the folks at the testing center are still wondered why anyone would show up to take a licensure exam in January while shivering with dripping wet hair.

The night before

" a student speaks

"The night before a test, I can't sleep. Then I worry because I can't sleep. Then I can't sleep because I'm worried that I won't be able to sleep. Then I worry about worrying that I'm worried that I can't sleep. By morning, I'm glad to get out of bed just to stop the terrible racket in my head."

— Marna Brohler, BSN student, Colorado

The night before the exam (a.k.a. "Exam Eve") is difficult for many students. Usually at about 5:30 PM. on Exam Eve, your brain reaches its final stuffing capacity. At that point, you may become fearful that your brain will short-circuit if you try to memorize another side effect of long-term milk of magnesia use. Since you don't want your brain to turn into a mass of quivering red jelly that refuses to produce anything on test day but the name of the dog you had in third grade, it's time to quit studying.

Pack your bag for the next day. Don't forget a couple of number-2 pencils, a snack, a watch, a sweatshirt, and other tools you need for the test. Pack earplugs if you need them and have already gotten approval for using them from the person who will be proctoring the exam. Make sure your car has gas, or that your bike tires have air, or that your personal dirigible has whatever it is that personal dirigibles need. If you take public transportation to school, make sure you have tokens and change.

After you've packed your bag, go outside and have some fun. You remember the concept of fun, don't you? Throw a Frisbee around with your best friend, lie under a tree and watch the squirrels play (join them if you're so inclined), go to a movie, or simply hang out with your kids.

The day of the exam

Before the exam begins

A few days before the exam, make sure you know where the exam is going to be held. Check the syllabus but double-check with the instructor (not another student) before the day of the exam.

Plan to get to the exam room about 15 minutes early. This will give you enough time to pick the most desirable test-taking location without having to be exposed to inordinate amounts of pre- testing mayhem in which fellow students grab you by the collar and gulp, "I . . . can't . . . believe . . . I . . . forgot . . . to . . . study . . . the . . . therapeutic . . . communication . . . techniques!"

Once you get to the room, scope out the scene for the chair that will work best for you. You might want to be on an aisle, or away from the door, or near an air-conditioning vent, or whatever is most sought after in your particular situation. Be alert for any environmental conditions that might distract from your ability to do your best on the exam. The school I attended for my associate's degree was owned by a hospital system that was spiraling into bankruptcy, and so a lot of "deferred maintenance" was practiced during our last semester. The seats most in demand during our final exam were located in a corner of the exam room where the ceiling tiles had already fallen in. This area was less likely to subject you to any of the brown ooze that seemed to drip perpetually from the remaining tiles.

If there is a chance that one of your more ethically challenged fellow students is going to want to do some cheating, sit very, very far away from them, in another time zone if possible. Schools of nursing deal out appropriately harsh measures to cheaters. In the midst of an exam, even if you're just telling a would-be cheater to "buzz off and get a life," the exam proctors have no way of knowing that and you can easily be implicated.

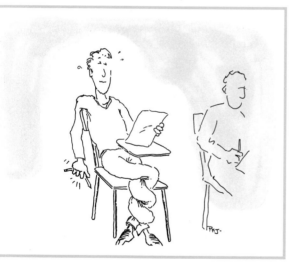

Try to eat something, even a small snack of complex carbohydrates, a few hours before the exam. If you feel too anxious or nauseated to eat, a sports electrolyte-replacement drink might work better for you, although drinking much before the exam will definitely increase the chances you will need to "use the facilities" during the exam.

Remember as you walk into the test that the wee bit of anxiety you may be experiencing is actually a positive thing. A small amount of anxiety can help you focus. You don't want to be too relaxed ("Hmm, oh look, it's the exam. This is one-third of my grade . . . oh, well . . . can't worry about it . . . what is it they say, 'hakuna matata' . . . I wonder if I have time for a little nap . . . .") or you won't be able to do your best work.

If you find yourself having a severe anxiety reaction, however, you'll want to review some of the methods for dealing with stress found in Chapter 2. For an exercise that is particularly good for test anxiety, see *Reducing stress with controlled breathing.*

Reducing Stress with
Controlled Breathing

An excellent way to reduce feelings of anxiety is to use the technique of controlled breathing (also called diaphragmatic breathing). When you control your breathing, you can break the pattern of shallow short breaths associated with anxious feelings. Deep abdominal or diaphragmatic breathing enhances the relaxation response. When a person exhales, tense muscles tend to relax. Diaphragmatic breathing causes the diaphragm to flatten and the abdomen to enlarge on inspiration. On exhalation, the abdominal muscles contract. As you slowly let out this deep breath, the other muscles of the body will tend to "let go" and relax. This technique enables you to breathe more deeply even if you just expand your chest on inspiration. Controlled breathing can be helpful to reduce anxious responses that occur at the beginning of the test, when stumped with a tough question, or when nearing the end of the test. During these critical times you can use controlled breathing to induce the relaxation response.

When practicing diaphragmatic breathing, place your hand slightly over the front of the lower ribs and upper abdomen so you can monitor the movement you're trying to achieve. As you become accomplished in this technique, you won't need to position your hands on the body. Practice the following steps:

1. Gently position your hands over the front of the lower ribs and upper abdomen.

2. Exhale gently and fully. Feel your ribs and abdomen sink inward toward the middle of the body.

3. Slowly inhale a deep breath through your nose, allowing the abdomen to expand first and then the chest. Do this as you slowly count to 4.

4. Hold your breath at the height of inhalation as you count to four.

5. Exhale fully by contracting the abdominal muscles and then the chest. Let all the air out slowly and smoothly through the mouth as you count to 8.

Monitor the pace of your breathing. Notice how your muscles relax each time you exhale. You may feel warm, tingly, and relaxed. Enjoy the feeling as you breathe deeply and evenly. You should practice this technique so that controlled breathing automatically induces the relaxation response after several breaths. Once you're able to induce the relaxation response with controlled breathing, you can effectively draw on this strategy when you need to be in control.

It is important not to do this exercise too forcefully or too rapidly because it can cause you to hyperventilate. Hyperventilation precipitates dizziness and lightheadedness. If either of these occur, cup your hands over your nose and mouth and slowly rebreathe your exhaled air. These symptoms should subside. Then, you can continue the exercise less vigorously. Always monitor your responses throughout the exercise.

Source: Reproduced with permission from: Patricia M. Nugent, *Test Success: Test-Taking Techniques for Beginning Nursing Students*. Philadelphia: F. A. Davis Co., 1997, p. 3. © 1997, the F. A. Davis Company.

Test-taking tips

READ THE DIRECTIONS

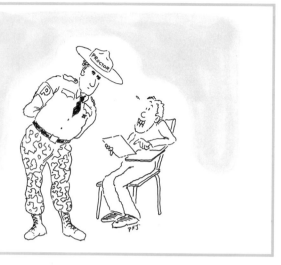

Our parents have been drilling this advice into our heads since we were old enough to read, but that doesn't make this advice any less valid. The instructions on the test you are taking are probably identical to those on every multiple-choice test you've ever taken in your whole life, but who knows? Maybe the instructor added a caveat such as, "Anyone willing to be a volunteer model for the next return demonstration on nasogastric tube insertions will be given 2 percentage points extra credit on this exam." You wouldn't want to miss that important information, would you?

Also, if you don't understand something on the exam, ask the proctor about it. The very worst the proctor can say is, "I'm sorry, I can't tell you that."

TIMING IS EVERYTHING

As soon as you take your place, synchronize your watch with the exam room clock. Besides making you feel like James Bond, this will give you the advantage of always having the "official" (proctor's) time on your desk so that you won't have to continually look up at the clock and get distracted by how many or few of your classmates have completed the exam.

Using the information you got from being a test sleuth, you already know roughly how many questions there are and how much time you have for the test, and thus how much time you can devote to each question. Once the proctor gives the signal to start, skim the test and answer the easy questions first to build your confidence, keeping in mind the time limit you have.

ELIMINATE ANSWERS TO IMPROVE THE ODDS

As you go through each question, first cross out any answers that make no sense. Second, look for answers that contradict basic nursing knowledge. Third, watch for answers that contain absolutes like "never" because these answers are seldom correct. Finally, pick the *best* answer based on which answer is *most* true. For example:

"Ms. Matilda Morris is a 2-day post-hip-replacement patient who asks for your help to change positions in bed. Which of the following would be an appropriate nursing intervention?

    A. Tell the patient she needs to change the position without your help. Never do for a patient what the patient can do for herself.
    B. Run screaming from the room.
    C. Explain to her that bed rest has been ordered and it will help her hip to heal better if she stays very still.
    D. Help her to reposition, keeping her hip in adduction.
    E. Help her to reposition, keeping her hip in abduction."

You can eliminate answer "B" immediately because there are very few situations in which it would be helpful for a nurse to scream and run away from a patient's room.

Answer "A" sounds somewhat plausible at the first read-through, because this answer is partially correct; modern nursing does encourage patients to be active participants in their own care. The tone of the answer (use of the words "tell the patient" rather than "encourage the patient") is a tip-off to continue to look for an answer that is more true.

Answer "C" contradicts basic nursing knowledge about the hazards of immobility.

The possible correct answers, then, are "D" or "E." If you remember what the proper position is for a patient's leg after hip replacement (abduction), then you know the correct answer is "E." What if your brain turns to marshmallow fluff and you can't remember the difference between abduction and adduction? Guess one of the two answers you still have left as viable choices. By the power vested in the process of elimination, you will have still increased your odds of getting the question correct to 50-50.

If you're completely stumped by a question, go back to the ABCs: What affects airway, breathing, and circulation the most? Finally, in the words of one BSN student who (wisely, I think) chose to remain anonymous: "If I had one piece of advice to give students to help get them through nursing school, I would tell them: If you don't know the answer, think Maslow and the hierarchy of needs. Remember that patient safety is always the number-one priority. Oh, and I would also tell them not to get Pavlov (the guy with the salivating dog) mixed up with Maslow. Nursing instructors don't like that at all."

ELIMINATE "DUMB" MISTAKES

Before you turn your masterpiece over to the exam proctor, look over each response quickly to make sure that you are actually answering the question asked. For example, make sure there are no questions in which you have chosen the answer to "All the following are nursing interventions for a patient with a broken big toe" when the actual question reads "All the following are nursing interventions for a patient with a broken big toe *except—*"

If the exam papers are graded by machine, check for stray marks that the machine might interpret as misplaced answers. Also, make sure that the little circle you meant to fill in for each answer is the circle that you actually filled in.

Troubleshooting test performance

" a student speaks

"I can't believe it. I've been getting 90s and above on all my exams in all my other classes and my prerequisites. Now I start my nursing classes and I'm barely passing. What happened??? Did I get stupid all of a sudden or what?"

— D.P., BSN student, New Mexico

Examine the problem for yourself

No one likes to do poorly on a test, and, in particular, no one likes to do poorly on a test when it seems one's entire future is determined by that test. So, if you find that you've not done as well as you would like on an exam, what's the next step?

If you've done well on exams in the past (and especially if you've done well on multiple-choice nursing exams), examine your pattern to see if you did anything differently this time. For example, perhaps you attended fewer lectures, or studied more from the notes and less from the book, or didn't review the older material as well as you usually do. If you feel fairly certain that you've identified the cause of your poor grade, simply resume your more successful pattern for the next test.

However, if you have done poorly on more than one test, or if you seem to know about the same amount of material as your study partners but consistently score lower on exams than they do, the problem may be more complicated.

Getting outside help

If you think you have a problem, the first thing I would advise is to make an appointment with your friendly neighborhood faculty member, preferably the faculty member who had the most input for the most recent test or who has given the most lectures. Make sure this person understands that you are coming to talk about how you can improve your test performance, not to complain about how crummy you think the test questions were (even if you think the test questions were indeed crummy).

I suggest making an appointment rather than just stopping by during office hours for two reasons. First, making an appointment gives the instructor a chance to think about how you can improve your performance. Perhaps the instructor has noticed that you always miss a particular kind of question, or that you are hesitant to ask a question in lecture if you are confused, or that it seems like you are always ill prepared for tests that take place on the morning after a full moon. These are patterns you might not have noticed, so pre-planned input can be vital here. Instructors may also be able to go over the test with you, or refer you to resources available in your school or community that assist students in developing test-taking skills or dealing with test anxiety.

Second, making an appointment demonstrates that you have good social skills and that how well you do on tests matters to you. Although we would hope that the meeting itself would be productive, if it isn't, you will still come out ahead because you have demonstrated these positive qualities to a faculty member. Call it trying to get "brownie points" if you want, but these are folks whom you may be asking to write recommendations for you in the future. Treating instructors with extreme courtesy (and even deference if required) is both appropriate and pragmatically smart.

A final word about grades

It's easy to get slightly (or extremely!) discouraged when we pour out our blood, sweat, and tears studying for exams and still only get grades that "squeak" us by to the next level. However, the ability to do well on multiple-choice exams and the ability to be an excellent nurse are not the same thing. As long as you are doing well in the clinical component of your courses, remember that "A" is not the only letter that equals "RN." A nursing school faculty member, who wishes to remain anonymous, told me this story:

"I had a student my first year of teaching who could never do well on the tests. She would get so anxious that she'd forget even her own name, I think! She always did well on the floor, but just barely passed her exams. She graduated, but certainly not with any honors, and I think it took her two tries to pass her boards. About 15 years later I had to go to the community hospital for some very painful surgery. The first night after surgery I was in bed, trying to sleep, and who should tiptoe in but that student, now an experienced RN! She took the best care of me of any of the nurses there, and I suspect I was a very demanding patient. In those moments, I was very glad she had persevered!"

So, squeakers, you've made it this far. Plug on!

RESOURCES

Web sites

MEDICAL MNEMONICS

www.medicalmnemonics.com/

This is just what the name says: a Web site devoted to col-
lecting all the useful (and not so useful) mnemonics that
students have developed over the years. Some of these will probably
be familiar to you; others you may never have thought about. This is
an attractive and quick-loading site. You can look for appropriate
mnemonics by browsing through clinical or pre-clinical disciplines,
or you can look them up alphabetically.

MIDDLE TENNESSEE STATE UNIVERSITY STUDENT SUCCESS SITE

www.mtsu.edu/~studskl/sucstu.html

If you want to know how successful students prepare for tests at
Middle Tennessee State University, this is the place to come. Don't
miss the cute graphics for much needed comic relief.

UNIVERSITY OF BUFFALO COUNSELING CENTER HOME PAGE

http://ub-counseling.buffalo.edu.stresstestanxiety.shtml

The friendly folks at the University of Buffalo Counseling Center developed this short and sweet guide to test anxiety that you may find
useful when exam time rolls around. It even details the physical
signs of test anxiety. As if we didn't already know!

UNIVERSITY OF CHICAGO STUDENT COUNSELING CENTER VIRTUAL PAMPHLET COLLECTION

www.uhs.bsd.uchicago.edu/scrs/vpc/

This collection of links to easy-to-read pamphlets put out by counseling services at the University of Chicago and many other universities is quick loading and unbelievably simple to use. It has a great section on tests, test taking, and studying as well as information about mastering test anxiety and doing well on multiple-choice tests. Don't miss the link to the "Certificate for the Right to Play."

CHAPTER **6**

Yes, You Can Avoid: Fatigue Related to Being Perceived as "Different"

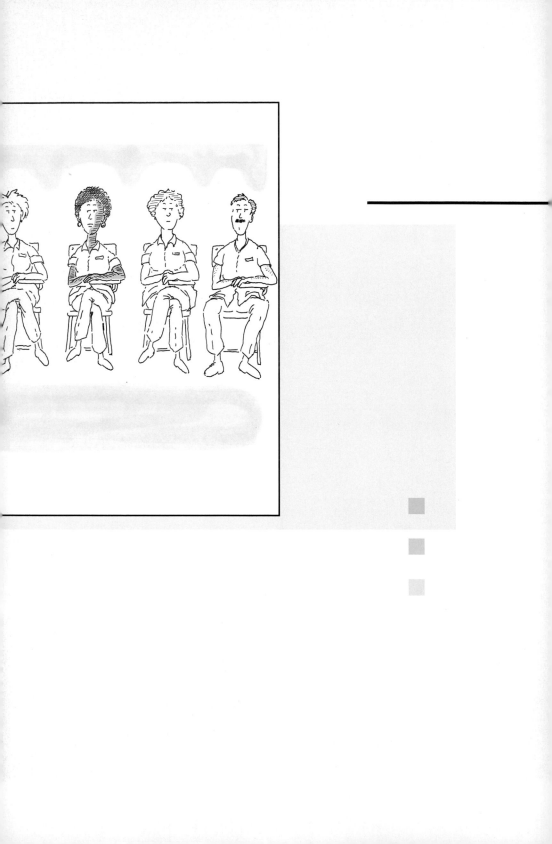

CHAPTER **6**

Yes, You Can Avoid: Fatigue Related to Being Perceived as "Different"

a student speaks

"I am a single mom with two school-age children, and going to nursing school has been the hardest thing I've ever done. I could not have done it, though, if my kids hadn't been so supportive. They really respect the time that my studies take. I feel guilty sometimes that they don't get much quality or quantity time with me."

— **Lisa Cohen, diploma student, Pennsylvania**

Nursing school is not easy for anyone. All students juggle complex demands and extraordinary workloads. They may also feel challenged in their nursing school career by encounters with people who are very different from themselves. This may include older students, male students, students in recovery from drug and alcohol addictions, students with disabilities, students who are non-native speakers of English, and sexual-minority students. A discussion of the challenges an individual in each of these groups might face in nursing school is unfortunately beyond the scope of this book, so I have chosen to include information about the diversity issues that were most frequently mentioned by the students I interviewed.

This chapter is intended to help nursing students who are of nontraditional age, or who are male, gay, lesbian, or bisexual, to deal with the challenges of nursing school. I hope that this chapter will also serve as a primer for other nursing students who wouldn't necessarily identify with these groups. By providing this information, I hope to help them understand what other nursing students (and coworkers and, ultimately, patients) may be dealing with in their lives.

If you are a nontraditional-age student

It probably goes without saying that not all nursing students today are dewy-eyed teen-age girls. Still, older people who enter nursing school may find themselves being looked at as if they had three heads. And that's not the only problem they face, especially if they're parents, single or otherwise.

Special time concerns for the older student

LEARNING THE FINE ART OF MULTITASKING

Students who have children say their time is their most valuable commodity. Many students told me that they are learning the art of multitasking and incorporating the whole family in their school projects. For example, one student said she got her preteens to quiz her on diseases of the digestive system while she drove them to school ("I got to gross *them* out for a change!"). Another said her partner served as her "guinea pig" whenever she needed to practice for her Physical Assessment class.

DROPPING YOUR STANDARDS A BIT

A second time saver older students mentioned was dropping your standards a little. At mealtime, your kids will probably like eating fast food once a week, and you can supplement it with easy-to-make veggies like baby carrots and celery sticks to ease your guilt. When they have friends over, tell them to pretend that it's the latest rage to have 6 months' dust accumulation on the furniture and infant-sized dustballs underneath the bed. Teach your kids how to separate their own laundry and then expect them to do it.

Explain to the kids that you can no longer provide transportation for every after-school activity ever invented. Have them choose the activity that means the most to them and explain that you will be the taxi for that activity but that they'll have to arrange alternative transportation for the rest. This will teach them negotiation skills and how to use available resources. However, make sure you double-check their chosen method of transportation! My grandma told my uncle he needed to find his own way home after his 4 days a week of play practice. On the play's opening night, she found he had been hopping the freight train to get home! For other tips on handling the multiple demands of school and family, see *When you also have a family.*

When You Also Have a Family

These tips were collected by Angela Pearch from a student nurse e-mail list, Future Nurses, based in Eugene, Oregon (*http://www.efn.org/~nurses/*).

- Lower your standard of housekeeping. You don't need to make the beds every day as long as your sheets are clean. You want the place to be clean enough to stay healthy and organized enough to find your shoes in the morning. Every thing else is just petty pride.

- Care and upkeep of a significant other are important. Tell your significant other how much you appreciate them and count on them. When they do something you find helpful, thank them. Remember, you're in this together.

- If you have all-day day care (not hourly), use it! Drop the kids off when the doors open and study. It helps the kids and you if you have a regular time when you pick them up, though.

- Shop around for reliable day care. Most facilities will send a child home "sick" with a touch of diarrhea or set an arbitrary temperature degree as the "sick" point. Have a back-up plan if your child is "under the weather."

- Look around your community for activities your kids can enjoy while you are in class or studying. Little League, after-school programs, and community events are all good possibilities.

- Set aside family time and protect it—even when you have a paper due the next day.

- Set aside study time and protect it—even if it means hiring a baby-sitter or trading baby-sitting duty with a friend.

- Enforce a "family homework time" and have everyone study together at the table. You will set an example of good study habits and have some extra family time, too.

CHOOSING A PROGRAM CAREFULLY

Parents and other nontraditional age students need flexibility in their schedules. Some schools are able to accommodate this, others aren't. To check for this, one single mother suggested, "When you have an entrance interview, say you are unavailable for the first time slot they offer you because you won't be able get a baby-sitter. If there is a long, awkward silence, you're almost guaranteed that few of the students have children. If they aren't able to accommodate you for an hour, think how inflexible the clinical schedules will be!"

Most programs allow you to take a part-time courseload, which sometimes works better with hectic work and child-care schedules.

EXAMINING YOUR OPTIONS

If you find yourself falling behind, you may feel that postponing school is the best option for you. However, a number of students cautioned against waiting for the perfect time to go to school, whether it be when your 4-year-old enters kindergarten, when your husband finishes his PhD, or when your 4-year-old finishes his PhD. Although there may be some times in your family's life span that are going to be more complicated than others, as one student said, "There is simply no good time for nursing school."

DEALING WITH A CHANGE IN STATUS

Although time-management strategies specific to the situation of a nontraditional-age student are important, the challenges of being an older student extend beyond searching for reliable day care or dealing with crayon marks on one's white clinical shoes. Most returning students have had successful careers and done just fine for many years without the advice of parents or teachers. Some respondents found it hard to adjust to the student role. Although this may be particularly true in the clinical arena, where students and faculty work most closely with one another, it can happen in the classroom also.

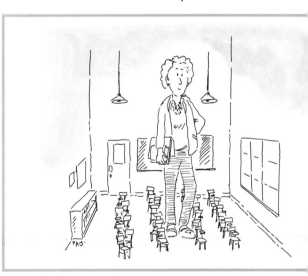

"I can't believe the silliness the instructors throw at us sometimes," said one 45-year-old associate degree student. "The other day they had a whole class on how to take good notes. If I didn't know how to take

profile

At age 56, Doris Weimar was dissatisfied with her job. "I was working [in a dead-end job] doing dumb things and getting angry because I was always in a role that was supporting people who had a college education. I was complaining in this manner to a friend, and she said, 'with all your complaints, why don't you do something?'"

"I countered with, 'I'm too old.' But my friend said, 'The time passes anyway.' I felt like someone had turned on the lights! While I was saying that I was too old [to go back to school], 20 years had passed. Right then I decided I couldn't say I was too old until I had given it my best shot."

Weimer remembers having her appendix out when she was 10 years old and observing the nurses as they ran up and down the wards taking care of patients. "For the first time I saw women moving with authority and competence instead of just sitting chained to a desk, " she explains. "They got to really think about something instead of just writing down someone else's thoughts. I declared then that I wanted to be a nurse, but my family was horrified. I even told my family about the cute outfits I had seen the nurses wearing." She adds, wryly, "It never occurred to me that their skin was probably rubbed raw from all the starch they had to use on their uniforms."

Encouraged by her friend's advice and inspired by her childhood memory, at the age of 56 Doris Weimar started her first semester of nursing school at a local community college. "I was sure that my 1944 high school education would be adequate," she said, "but when I got there, doing my prerequisite classes and my nursing classes at the same time . . . well, it was quite intense."

But Weimar persevered. After finishing her associate's degree, she worked as a staff nurse, and she completed her BSN when she was well into her 60s. "My goal was to eventually go into psych nursing because I thought I could make a difference there," she says. She attained her goal, working in an inpatient psychiatric facility.

After a number of years, Weimar retired. However, not long after, a local university was expanding their nursing programs and needed the nursing lab reconstructed. They thought she was the perfect person for the job. So, 7 months into her retirement—when others her age might aspire only to sipping tropical drinks around a pool in Miami Beach—she became director of the Learning Resource Center (LRC) at Temple University.

It was a task Weimar tackled with matter-of-fact enthusiasm. "I believe the basis for any good nursing education is not how many credits you amass, but how good you are at basic assessments," she says. "So, eventually I ended up redesigning the whole lab so that it was pretty as well as functional. For example, I wanted an [examination] table for each partner. When I was in school, we learned our assessment skills in a chair—but it's not the best way to learn. I became very resourceful in finding creative ways to acquire needed equipment because I wanted to make sure that students had everything I could have used as a student that wasn't there. We expanded the hours the lab was open and invited the students to form groups and come for practice. Instead of seeing it as a punishment, students came to treasure their time in the lab."

"Some of the moments I valued most were teaching students the nursing process," she explains. "When you have a student whose thoughts are beginning to fly like bats around their head, using the nursing process slows them down and identifies what they need to do and where they need to go."

Weimar has retired a second time, but her love for nursing and educating future nurses is still a part of her life. She tutors students who didn't pass the NCLEX on the first try, evaluating their strengths and weakness and addressing them in a systematic fashion. "When a student is really struggling," she says, "I find that nine times out of ten they are trying to memorize their way through the material. The trick is to quickly get them into critical thinking. I find that the concepts just need to penetrate. Often, all a student needs to succeed is to store up some success and feel confident in what they are doing."

---

good notes, I'd look it up on the Internet or find a book or something. I hate having my time wasted like that!"

Students had very few sure-fire strategies for handling the discomfort that comes with the sudden relegation to student status. Some said they simply ignored the slights and focused their energy on their studies; others suggested that older students should communicate openly with instructors about their expectation to be treated like adults. One student had been a manager of a large hardware store until he started nursing school. He said that one instructor talked to him in a way he considered condescending. When he mentioned it to her, he said, "She apologized and explained that she had taught for many years when the only students were 18-year-old females who had never lived anywhere but in their parents' homes. She explained that nursing education was a changing world and she was not changing as quickly as it was. I really appreciated her candor, and we understood each other better after that."

FACING THE COMPLEXITIES OF RELATIONSHIPS

Many nontraditional-age students said that going to nursing school dealt a rather harsh blow to their primary relationships. "Beware of letting the fact that you are in school become the scapegoat for all that is wrong in the relationship," cautioned Carla Gomez, whose 10-year marriage survived nursing school "only with a lot of really long talks and a great deal of compromise." In other words, nursing school might be responsible for the fact that the kids are a week late for their 6-month dental checkup, but probably not for the fact that your partner thinks your mother smells of mothballs and meddles too much in your personal financial affairs.

Interestingly, although many students felt that their primary relationships were affected negatively by the time they spent on their studies, more than a few nurse-educators said they had seen a fair number of negative relationships dealt a fatal blow by one partner's experience in nursing school. "We should call nursing school 'Get Out of an Abusive Relationship School,'" said one nursing instructor from the Midwest. "It's amazing to watch middle-aged women make better decisions as their self-esteem and earning power grow and they realize they don't have to depend on someone who hurts them."

If you are a student who is gay, lesbian, or bisexual

" a student speaks

"When I was an undergraduate, my professor was showing a movie called *Future Shock*. During the video two gay men were getting married. My entire class started laughing. I felt humiliated and degraded by their laughter. I decided to leave the room. I had two choices, to exit using the door at the back of the class or to use the door at the front of the class. I picked up my books, walked to the front of the class, jerked open the door, and slammed the door behind me. As I stood in the hallway crying, I noticed the laughter had immediately stopped. Nothing was ever said to me about my behavior that day. At that time in my life I did not have what it takes to defend my culture against such an insult."

— W.H., FNP student, Mississippi

In the close-knit communities of nursing school, many sexual-minority students are afraid to discuss their closest relationships for fear of how their peers will react. One student who attended a BSN program in Texas said, "In my Health Assessment class we sometimes had to get partially undressed to practice certain aspects of the physical exam. One day before class a bunch of students were talking about another student in the class and saying 'Oh, I'd never get undressed in front of her, she's such a lezzie,' and laughing. I didn't know what to say. When my partner of 3 years broke up with me the night before the final exam, you can bet I made up a quick story about having allergies when those students asked me why my eyes were red. They would have been really mad if they knew they had undressed in front of a real, live lesbian all semester long."

Yet some students say they are able to be open about their sexual orientation and found that it has helped, rather than hindered, their nursing school career. I talked with one student who attended an associate degree program in upstate New York and struggled to continue her work as a lay midwife for the Amish, raise a 13-year-old son, and take care of her partner, who was dying of cancer. She said that being out about her sexual orientation "was positive because it allowed me to get support . . . and talk about my family concerns."

Sexual-minority students urge prospective students to consider whether a school is gay-friendly when they make their admission decision. They can ask about the school's reputation at the local gay community center or inquire about the existence of a gay support group at the office of student life. "Nursing school is too hard to be trying to hide all the time," said one gay male student who attended an associate degree program in the urban Southwest. "Sure, my classmates don't have to know all my business, but I'm open about my sexuality because I don't want to be the only one during study breaks who's not sharing what I did over the winter holiday."

Sometimes other students assume a fellow student's sexual orientation because of that student's appearance or mannerisms. Often this is because the individual looks different from and displays mannerisms not traditionally associated with their gender. "People assume I'm a lesbian because I wear my hair very short and never wear makeup," said one student from New York, "And they're right . . . I am, in fact, a lesbian. But what they don't know is that I have a classmate who has long blonde hair and wears a skirt to every class . . . and she's a lesbian, too!" It is important for nursing students to realize that the gender presentation of an individual is completely separate from their sexual orientation. Individuals who have what society might consider a "nonmainstream gender expression" may self-identify as gay, lesbian, bisexual, or heterosexual, or might feel that none of these labels fit their sexual orientation. Many individuals who have transitioned or are in the process of transitioning (i.e., changing their appearance and body to match their internal gender identity, sometimes through hormones and surgery) experience discrimination at school, in the workplace, and when seeking health care. For one striking example of this discrimination, see *In memoriam: Tyra Hunter*. More information about how to be supportive of fellow students, colleagues, and patients who may be dealing with gender issues can be found in the Resources section at the end of this chapter.

In Memoriam: Tyra Hunter

Tyra Hunter, a young transgender woman in Washington, was struck in a hit-and-run auto accident on August 7, 1995. EMS technicians were called to the scene and began treating her. Her injuries were extremely severe, and her survival was uncertain. In the course of her treatment, an EMS technician cut open her pants and discovered she had a penis, whereupon he backed away; began making jokes about the prostrate, bleeding woman; and refused to render further treatment. Unmoved by pleading bystanders—including one who yelled out, "It don't make any difference, he's [sic] a person, he's a human being"—the EMS technician allowed Tyra to lie on the pavement untended for 3 to 5 minutes. An EMS supervisor finally came to Tyra's aid. She died later at a local hospital. More than 2000 people attended her funeral.

Source: From GenderPAC (Gender Public Advocacy Coalition), New York, NY

If you are a male student

" a student speaks

"I've never been a minority before, and I've found that I'm not a very good sport about it. Sometimes I felt like saying with a fake hurt tone, 'I am not an animal. I am a human being,' because it seems like all the women were treating me like I was a part of a different species or something."

— M.L., BSN student, Kentucky

Special considerations in choosing a school

In e-mails and interviews, male nursing students consistently told

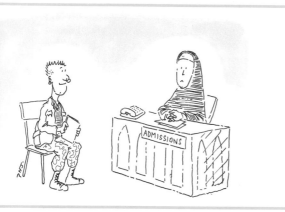

me that it is important to find an environment in which male students are treated as quite literally "one of the guys," not some kind of aberration from the norm, that is, a female nursing student. "Shop around," said one student. "I am 6 foot 4 inches tall, wear my hair in a modified flat top, and have multiple piercings and tattoos. When I went for an admission interview at the local Catholic university, I knew it was not the place for me. The nun who was interviewing me looked like she was afraid I would steal her purse."

Students suggested that, during the application process, prospective students visit the campus and talk to male students. They said that one student can be someone the administration selects to meet with you, but that you should also talk to at least one other student whom you approach in the cafeteria or after a class. "Just ask directly," said one student, "is this a good place for a nursing student who happens to be male?"

What does it mean to be male in a female environment?

Male students say their nursing school experience has taught them how similar and how dissimilar the experiences of men and women are. One student said he was amazed by an older instructor who in class always referred to the doctor as "he" and the nurse as "she." "I was offended because a hypothetical nurse can be either he or she," the student explains, "but then I thought, women are being slighted by this also. Who says a hypothetical doctor has to be male?"

Other students said they learned a great deal about their attitudes to-ward women and power during their nursing school career. "I thought I was a liberated man and sensitive to women and all that," said one student, "but I found out I needed to grow up a lot when I found myself chafing at women in leadership roles. All I have to say is 'Guys, resolve your issues with women (especially your mother!) before you start school.'"

Handling being treated differently

ON THE LABOR AND DELIVERY FLOOR

The area in which the most male students expressed concern about being able to participate fully was in the labor and delivery clinical rotation. Traditionally, labor and delivery have been very female dominated, and male nursing students said some people with whom they had contact, most often the staff at the site of their clinical rotation, expressed concerns about having males on the floor. One male BSN student said, "The day I was supposed to go for a delivery, the floor nurse asked the patient—while I was standing in the room—'You don't want a male student, do you?' Of course the patient said no. What else was she going to say at that point?" If they didn't want to settle for watching patient instruction videos in the lounge, male students said they needed to be assertive and have a good relationship with the clinical instructor to gain access to an actual labor and delivery experience.

"My instructor and I always assumed there would be no problem, and so there wasn't," another student said. "The first delivery I was supposed to observe didn't want a student at all, so it wasn't really a problem with me in particular. At the second delivery, they were very glad to have a student there because I focused all my energies on the dad, who was a nervous wreck. I talked with him about my rela-

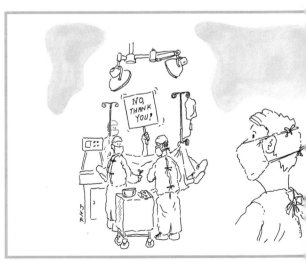

tionship with my children and even had to coach him on his breathing at one point. He was really nervous!"

One associate degree student said, "I love that scene in [the television show] *ER* where that nurse tells the doc that he's a trained professional colleague and that he doesn't want to be used as a security guard. I think I actually got up on my couch and cheered when I saw that. I feel frustrated when I'm treated as Mr. Brawny or always get called away from my patient to do the heavy lifting someplace else. I think someone needs to do some research on male nurses and back injuries. We end up using our backs all the time."

To mitigate the effects of this "Mr. Brawny syndrome," students suggested politely explaining one's role—"I'm a nursing student. I'm

Are You One of Those Male Nurses?

Nursing students who happen to be male are often cross-examined by patients, families, and staff alike. Here are three questions that male nursing students told me they are frequently asked—and some responses they have formulated. (Use at your own risk.)

ARE YOU A MALE NURSE?

"Yes."

"Yes, I'm a nursing student and yes, I am a male."

"Hmm, oh yeah." (One student said, "I've heard this question so much it doesn't even register any more.")

ARE YOU GAY?

"No."

"Yes."

"No, and you?"

"Yes, and you?"

"Kind of a private question, don't you think?"

"I don't usually find it necessary to discuss my sexual orientation with patients in order to give them good care."

WEREN'T YOU SMART ENOUGH TO BE A DOCTOR?

"Of course I am, but I wanted to be a nurse."

"I thought nurses' uniforms were much more fetching."

"I tried being a doctor, but it was boring because they don't have enough to do."

glad to help out, but for today my primary responsibility is . . . "—and talking to the clinical instructor about the situation. One student said that when he approached his instructor about having his work constantly interrupted with requests for lifting assistance, she was very understanding and said she had tried to educate the staff on this particular floor but was having difficulty. "Finally," the student said, "she suggested that I tell the staff I had an old back injury and couldn't lift more than 35 pounds. I don't know why they didn't question that I suddenly developed an old back injury halfway through the semester. Anyway, it worked."

Male students reported that, no matter where they did their clinical rotations, they were asked the same questions. For these questions, and some responses the students suggested, see *Are you one of those male nurses?*

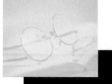

RESOURCES

Web sites

AMERICAN ASSOCIATION FOR MEN IN NURSING HOME PAGE

http://aamn.freeyellow.com/

This site includes resources and information about membership (open to women as well as men) and the AAMN's annual convention.

ASSOCIATION FOR NON-TRADITIONAL STUDENTS IN HIGHER EDUCATION

www.antshe.org/

ANTSHE is an international partnership of students, academic professionals, institutions, and organizations whose mission is to encourage and coordinate support, education, and advocacy for the adult learning community. This site contains articles and excellent links.

BACK TO COLLEGE WEB PORTAL

http://www.back2college.com/

This site's motto should be "before you go back to school, go to this site." All the information you might possibly need about returning to school and then some is here. You can sign up for a free newsletter here, use the curriculum finder to locate a school or program that fits your needs, peruse the information about financial aid for returning students, or follow links to numerous online tutoring sites.

CANADIAN MEDICAL ASSOCIATION JOURNAL: "NOT ALL YOUR PATIENTS ARE STRAIGHT"

www.cma.ca/cmaj/vol-159/issue-4/0370.htm

This is an excellent article about providing care for people in the lesbian, gay, bisexual, and transgender communities. It uses real-life examples and covers care issues across the life span.

GAY HEALTH HOME PAGE

www.gayhealth.com

This site contains information about health care for lesbian, gay, bisexual, and transgendered people as well as a provider's forum for gay, lesbian, bisexual, and transgendered healthcare providers. The provider's forum is new but looks promising, with multiple articles, threaded discussions, and an e-mail newsletter available.

GENDER PAC HOME PAGE

www.gpac.org

This is the home page of the Gender Public Advocacy Coalition. Read here about gender expression and health care.

MEN IN AMERICAN NURSING HISTORY

www.geocities.com/Athens/Forum/6011/index.html

This is an illustrated trip through the history of men in nursing in the United States. Although it hasn't been updated recently, it contains many fascinating photos you won't want to miss, displayed on an interesting yellow background.

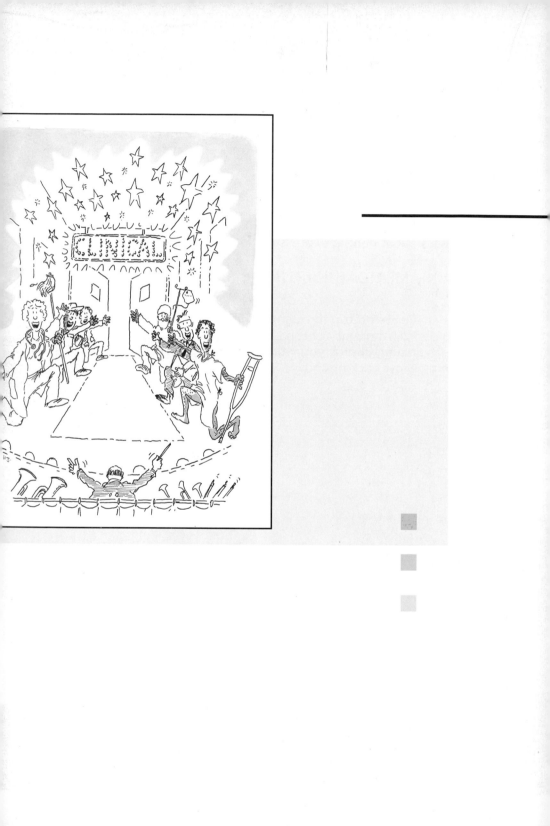

CHAPTER 7

Yes, You Can Avoid: Fear Related to the Start of Clinical Rotations

" a student speaks

"Clinical was different than any other experience I've had. I felt like I was all thumbs for the first few weeks, but now, looking back, I was doing just fine. One of the most amazing things is how forgiving patients can be. My very first clinical day, I was assigned to an older man from Colombia who spoke almost no English. Luckily, one of my classmates had a Spanish-English dictionary. We communicated with that and by pointing and hand signs. He was so good natured about the whole thing, it gave me the courage to come back the next clinical day."

— P.P., AD graduate, Pennsylvania

If you are a new nursing student anticipating clinical and your first hands-on experience in caring for patients, butterflies may already be partying in your stomach. You may have heard about clinical instructors with hair-trigger tempers, overworked staff nurses, impatient patients, and uniforms that scare the children when you do pediatrics rotations.

Much of this is true. Welcome to nursing.

But, remember, this is only the bad news. The good news is that you will have the satisfaction and privilege of helping people at some of the most vulnerable times of their lives.

Choosing a clinical instructor

a student speaks

"[Clinical experiences] that are not helpful include rotations on a floor that feels resentful toward students. Although the resentment can be an individual thing, I've found that in some areas at our particular hospital there was a predominantly anti-student attitude among the staff. I also found it wise to listen to what other students said from previous experiences/knowledge. That helped me decide which areas I would try to avoid. Sometimes, of course, you can't help which rotation you get. If you get a lemon, then you just have to make lemonade."

— Jenny Smith, AD graduate, Oregon

In many schools, students have no choice about who they have for a clinical instructor. If your school has some mechanism for allowing you to choose your clinical instructor, you should talk with students in the class before yours to get the lowdown on each one. Get their perceptions of each instructor's skills, fairness, and flexibility. Make sure you talk with a number of students to get a balanced view.

Ideally, schools will place instructors only on floors where they have extensive experience. However, as you may have noticed, nursing school conditions are sometimes less than ideal. Ask other students and your academic adviser about the experience and specialization of potential clinical instructors. If your instructor is a psych nurse teaching the ICU rotation or an ICU nurse teaching in the incarcerated juvenile psych ward, you may be able to muddle through together, but you will probably not have the learning experience you are looking for.

Also, be aware that although a certain instructor may have a reputation as being tough, it doesn't necessarily mean you need to avoid them like the bubonic plague. Some instructors are demanding but fair, and you may learn more from that instructor than from one who doesn't require as much work or preparation. Again, students who have already had this instructor can give you their insights. Ask individual students for their opinions, away from other students. It may seem simplest to ask a group of students waiting for exams to be posted, "Hey, what did you guys think of Ms. Weatherbee when you had her for clinical?" However, it's pretty much open season on clinical instructors when nursing students get together. Few will want to publicly admit that Ms. Weatherbee, who has a reputation for being a battle-ax, taught them more about pediatric oncology than they had ever hoped to know.

Choosing a clinical site

Like your clinical instructor, your clinical site may be left up to the luck of the draw and the whim of the nursing school gods. However, if you do have some options, try to research the facilities offered as much as you can.

First of all, try to ascertain whether the clinical site welcomes students. It's a rare clinical site that places a flashing neon sign located just outside the elevator that warns, "All nursing students are kindly asked to go away. We do not want you here." However, based on information you've gleaned from other students, friends you may have who work at different hospitals or institutions, and your own detective work, you can figure out which sites should have such a sign posted! Some floors may have too many patients per nurse for staff nurses to spend any meaningful time with students, especially during the first semester, when it's customary to spend more time spilling bedpans and losing thermometers than actually providing patient care.

On other floors, there may be ongoing conflict between the floor nurses and the nurse managers, or between different shifts. In these cases, the needs of students for clear guidance can be lost in the shuffle. Finally, if the entire institution is in some type of conflict or difficulty (such as a labor dispute, reorganization, or extensive lay-offs), the staff will probably have little energy to do anything other than maintain their workload and try and provide the best patient care they can. In today's nursing climate, it may be difficult to find a clinical site that is not undergoing some kind of internal upheaval. With an aware, supportive instructor, rotating through these floors may even be a good learning experience. However, it is best to avoid sites with problems like these in your first clinical rotation.

Outfitting yourself for clinicals

Uniforms

Many nursing school uniforms are rivaled only by nun habits for their impracticality and odd appearance. At my school, the associate degree program's uniform consisted of polyester double-knit white pants with a white zipper-front shirt and a blue-and-white-striped snap-up blouse. We made quite a sensation when we rode the sub-ways to and from clinical. Small children asked us if we were dentists, and the local high school kids called us everything from Brady Bunch rejects to Amazon Smurfs. Jessica Wheeler, a BSN student in Connecticut, said her school's uniform consists of ". . . white pants that are awful; they have an elastic waist and are very see-through. We also have to wear a white scrub shirt and a blue lab coat that has our name and school on it. The pants are not comfortable at all."

No one knows quite why many student nurse uniforms are so bizarre (if you want to hear a really scary story, ask someone who graduated from nursing school 30 years ago about the black-stocking days), but they are purposely designed to look different from what the staff nurses wear. This, believe it or not, is to our advantage. It prevents first-semester students from being handed the ambu bag in the middle of a full code by a resident who mistakenly believes the student is an experienced, licensed nurse.

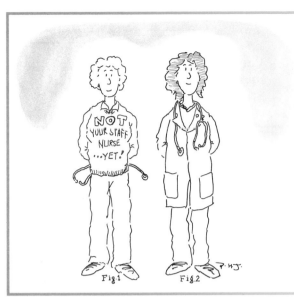

Some programs allow students to wear white scrubs with some identifying mark, such as an embroidered school insignia or school patch. If your school is one of these, count your blessings every clinical day and skip the rest of this section. If your school is not so enlightened, don't despair. There are ways to ameliorate the effects of even the most humiliating or uncomfortable uniform.

First, you may be able to get away with your own mini-modifications. These are least likely to be noticed if they affect comfort rather than appearance. For example, 4 weeks into my first clinical rotation, I thought that perhaps no one would care if I substituted a white cotton T-shirt for the polyester zipper front shirt that we had to wear. Because I still wore the striped blue "Smurf" blouse on top, no one ever said anything, and I was much happier with cotton instead of double-knit polyester against my skin. You may be able to get away with substituting nearly identical pants that are made of a comfortable material instead of something that gives you a rash. It all depends on how interested the clinical instructor is in identical uniforms and how much pressure there is from the school to make sure everyone conforms to the letter of the dress code. The first few times you try a substitution, you may want to bring along the actual uniform piece so you can change back in case the clinical instructor threatens to send you home or take off points from your clinical grade.

Second, you may find that there is some flexibility about the uniform, although it may not be in writing. For example, on one floor where I had clinical, we had many patients who were in isolation. The combination of wearing stifling plastic barrier gowns over our polyester uniforms left us emerging from our patients' rooms looking like lost sea otters. After watching one student struggle valiantly to avoid dripping perspiration into a sterile field while changing a dressing, our instructor emerged from the patient's room, called a quick conference, and announced, "Don't quote me on this, but please wear cotton scrubs from now on."

If your uniform is too impractical for your clinical situation, try approaching the instructor about modifying it in some way. You'll want to have this conversation privately and off the floor, and preferably not at the end of a long clinical day when you both are craving a caffeinated beverage and a nap. There's always the risk that the instructor may say, "You need to take it up with the program director/dean/board of directors," which may or may not be a viable option depending on the time and energy you have and how much you actually care. If the uniform is really scary, you can consider any work you do toward getting it modified to be an act of loving service for the future generations of nursing students at your school.

Be forewarned—if you try to make a case for modifying the uniform and your plea is rejected, your adherence to the dress code may be watched very carefully for the rest of your nursing school career. You should be prepared to endure wearing every snap and button of the prescribed uniform.

Equipment

When you start buying equipment for clinical, it's easy to overspend because there is such a vast array of potentially useful stuff available. However, your school will probably help you out by providing a list of suggested equipment and recommended vendors. Some schools require students to purchase a bag of equipment that is used for both lab and clinical, which might include IV bags, catheter kits, reflex hammer, and a penlight.

As for other equipment, no matter what the guy in the school bookstore or medical supply shop tries to tell you, you don't need a $150 cardiac stethoscope. Nobody expects you to identify and grade heart murmurs your first day on the floor anyway. As long as your stethoscope is serviceable for hearing bowel sounds, hearing breath sounds, and taking an apical pulse, it will work for at least the first year. On the other hand, don't buy the $5.95 generic stethoscope that looks (and sounds) as if it came out of a cereal box. A good rule of thumb is that if you find yourself writing "lung sounds decreased all fields" on more than a few notes in a row, it's probably time to up-grade your stethoscope. Or possibly clean out the earpieces.

You will need some other basic things for almost every clinical experience. These include a watch with a second hand, a couple of black pens (or a dozen if you're like me and tend to leave a trail of pens behind you wherever you go), a penlight, a calculator, goggles with sidepieces, bandage scissors, and very comfortable shoes.

There are also plenty of references you can purchase to help you out at clinical, and the guy at the bookstore (and your instructors) will probably suggest a number of them. The bare basics include some kind of drug guide and a pocket-sized clinical procedures handbook that you can use to refresh your memory when your mind suddenly goes blank about how to mix regular and long-acting insulin.

For references beyond the basics, team up with your fellow students and have one person bring the medical/surgical book, another a lab handbook, and so on. The folks on the subway who've been bruised by the loaded bookbags of nursing students on their way to clinical will benefit, and so will your back and your backpack.

Preparation

Getting lab experience

" a student speaks

"Clinical skills labs definitely help, especially if things are set up basically the same as the hospital where you're going to be doing your clinicals; for example, if they have similar equipment. I was so glad our skills lab used the same equipment as the hospital. If you have the time, go back to the lab and practice, practice, practice with the equipment. It's much better than totally embarrassing yourself or getting extremely frustrated while doing

patient care. Things like clearing pumps, changing PCA [patient-controlled analgesia] vials, IV tube changes, etc. can all cause much unneeded stress in clinical. So there really is a good reason for having those things there for you in lab. It's a gold mine if you choose to look at it that way."
— **Jenny Smith, AD graduate, Oregon**

The time I've spent in the nursing lab has been either a completely useless torture or the best thing since automatic IV pumps, depending on what kind of equipment was available and, more important, whether we spent more time listening to an instructor or engaged in hands-on practice.

Nursing instructors everywhere love showing those videos that demonstrate clinical skills. But it seems that most nursing students despise them. This is probably because nursing school is one long sleep-deprivation experiment, and we are incapable of learning anything with the lights turned low because we instantly slip into dreamland. But until nursing instructors get the message and offer an alternative, you need to make the most of the video learning experience. Probably the best thing to help you stay awake is actually to do any assigned reading related to the videos. Having even a smattering of knowledge will make the subject seem more interesting to you as well as make more sense. Not only that, you can try to guess the next action of the folks in the video—for example, what the next step is in doing the bed-bath. This makes video watching an active rather

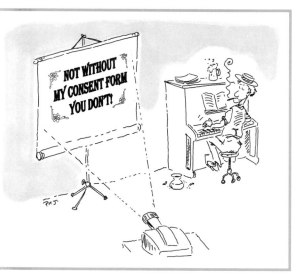

NOT WITHOUT MY CONSENT FORM YOU DON'T!

than passive learning experience. If all else fails, take painstakingly detailed notes. This will keep you awake, you'll have information about the video to refer to later, and the instructor will be impressed by your diligence (and it never hurts to impress an instructor!).

Most nursing labs have mannequins that are used for demonstrating and practicing different procedures. Unfortunately, no matter how much money your school has spent on mannequins and no matter how technically and anatomically correct they are, providing care for a mannequin bears almost no resemblance to providing care for a real patient. The behavior of a mannequin is predictable, whereas the behavior of a living, breathing patient is not. Still, mannequins can provide a practice field to help you develop your ability to do typical nursing procedures (such as tube feedings, IM injections, or wound care) and can bolster your confidence when you face a real patient.

After you practice your skills, the next step is usually an assessment of your ability to perform those skills, commonly called a return demonstration. Many students (myself included) find return demonstrations stressful no matter how much they've practiced. I flunked my vital signs return demonstration because my hands were shaking so badly I couldn't hold the stethoscope still enough to hear anything. I was devastated at the idea of coming back the next week to try again, but the lab instructor was a compassionate soul; she gave me a hug and said, "You'll get it next time. And when you pass your boards you'll look back on this and laugh." She was right on both counts, although I certainly didn't believe her at the time. You may find the stress-busting techniques in Chapter 2 helpful in dealing with return demonstrations. Also, talk about your feelings with your classmates. You may be surprised to find that they are as nervous as you are. Finally, remember that return demonstrations are a tool designed to help your instructors assess your knowledge and ability to perform clinical skills safely. Thinking of the situation as a learning experience may help reduce some of your anxiety.

Getting the most out of clinical orientation

Your clinical orientation will also help you prepare for your clinical experiences. Since you will probably have a limited amount of time to be oriented to the clinical site, make the most of the time you do have by asking many questions. If you don't understand something, ask. If you still don't understand something, ask again. Your instructors may have been through the clinical orientation a thousand times, so it's up to you to remind them that this is your first.

Sometimes instructors have a list of things for students to find (like a scavenger hunt) during the orientation time. If such a list is not provided, prepare your own, and keep asking where things are until you get answers. Some things you should know about each clinical site you rotate through include: location of fire doors; fire procedures, and location of fire-control equipment; how to get help in case of a patient emergency; and the location of emergency equipment. It also helps to know where to find the dirty and clean linen, policy and procedure book, extra forms, bath supplies, and comfort items for patients. Finally, make sure you know the location of the patient kitchen as well as the staff bathroom, because, as Jenny Smith, an AD graduate from Oregon points out, "You'll never know when you might need to throw up."

Managing pre-clinical paperwork

a student speaks

"[For our prep sheets] we had to have the name of the patient, the diagnosis, pathophysiology of the diagnosis, medications, side effects, effect of disease on person, nursing diagnosis (gag!). We had two care plans per rotation and a couple of teaching plans and, oh, then there was the focused function assessment. It contained 50 million questions that you were supposed to get from the patient based on Gordon's functional health patterns. [You'd be taking care of] an 80-year-old lady status post a bowel resection, and you were supposed to slip in the 'Are you sexually active and do you do breast exams' question while you did the bedbath or something. Those were ridiculous. Most of the clinical work was helpful in the beginning and then extremely excessive."

— **Laura Baker, BSN graduate, New York**

One of the most challenging aspects of clinical rotations is managing the pre-clinical paperwork in the small amount of time given you to complete it. If you can swing it at all, try to get off from your job on the night before clinical (especially in the beginning of your rotations). If you can, arrange for child care so that you can look up the nursing interventions for a patient with a total hip replacement without dealing with constant requests for a peanut-butter-and-toothpaste sandwich or permission to give the dog a haircut or whatever your kids tend to ask for when they know you're otherwise involved.

During your initial meeting with your instructors, make sure you understand exactly what their expectations are regarding written paperwork. For example, do they want a care plan turned in for each patient every clinical day? Do they expect you to make up drug cards, or can you use the ones that came with your drug guide? Do they prefer the care plans to be word-processed? Typed? Scripted in calligraphy on purple construction paper?

Most nursing students I talked with said that for each patient they were going to take care of in clinical, they at least had to look up the patient's admitting diagnosis, history, medications, interventions and assessments to be performed on the patient, and then come up with nursing diagnoses and rationales with interventions. This seems like a lot of work, and it is very time consuming. However, if you can concentrate while you're completing the paperwork and think about the disease process and the way it relates to the assessments and nursing interventions you will perform, you'll be honing your nursing process skills as well as preparing for the immediate care you'll be giving the next day.

A final note about care plans

Some nursing programs put a great deal of emphasis on writing care plans; others emphasize different methods for teaching the nursing process. If you have to do a bunch of care plans during clinical rotations, it's tempting to "borrow" your care plans from one of the many care plan books available. This will, of course, decrease your workload, but it will defeat the whole purpose of doing care plans, which is to help you learn to think your way through the nursing process—a skill that's needed to pass the NCLEX. There are a number of good books and Web sites that can help you get started with your care plans (some are included in the Resources section at the end of this chapter), but copying a plan verbatim out of a book is a waste of time for all involved.

The night before

As the panic builds, remember that the nursing school curriculum is designed to prepare you before you even set foot in the hospital. By the time clinical starts, you should have had at least a few days in the lab learning about tube safety, body mechanics, and personal care. You will have had basic CPR training. In short, you should have all the basic tools you need for you (and your patient) to survive your first day on the floor.

Of course, no matter how well prepared you are, you will feel some anxiety as the start of clinical approaches. If you have concerns about your preparation, ask your lab instructor. Unless this is the first time they have taught Bedpans and Siderails 101, they've undoubtedly heard concerns like yours before. They may be able to give you pointers to help with some of your clinical skills or perhaps even a pep talk to boost your confidence.

Once you get down to the night before your first clinical, however, you will probably wonder why you ever started nursing school in the first place. You may develop a stomachache, backache, or headache. You may have a fight with your spouse over not wiping off the top of the ketchup bottle. You may think that the cat is intentionally stomping across the carpeted floor just to annoy you. All this is very normal.

If you have a friend, sister, mother, father, third cousin or stepaunt who is a nurse, now is the time to have a heart-to-heart talk with them. Usually a simple "How did you feel before your first day on the hospital floor?" is sufficient. Experienced nurses love to talk about how they got sick every hour on the hour the whole night before their first clinical day. It reminds them of how far they've come, and it will remind you that you're not alone.

If you are still feeling uptight, resign yourself to it—don't add insult to injury by being anxious about being anxious. Use this anxiety to help you prepare more completely, spend some time visualizing yourself having a great day, then try to get a good night's sleep. Remember, a moderate amount of anxiety means you have the proper respect for the task you are about to undertake. Tomorrow you will be walking into a room that contains a real patient with a real health problem who is struggling through a vulnerable point in their life. It's a good thing to retain a sense of awe at our involvement. For one student's account of this experience see *"They should have sent a poet."*

"They Should Have Sent a Poet"

My dad sent me an e-mail last week that ended, "Well, Cheri, your grand-dad used to say that if every day you see the sunrise and sunset, you work a little, you laugh a lot, and you sleep well, close to the people you love, you can count yourself successful." I saw the sun coming up as I walked to the hospital Wednesday morning, as I do most clinical days. And over the next 8 hours, I saw two babies born. I don't care about nurses becoming immune to emotion. God help me if I ever witness something like that again and don't have tears fogging my glasses and the lump in my throat that I had this week. All I could think of was what Jodie Foster kept saying in the movie *Contact*: "They should have sent a poet . . . I had no idea."

One second there were 9 people in the room, the next there were 10. It was better than the Grand Canyon, the Statue of Liberty, a rainbow, the Rangers winning the World Series, and college graduation put together.

I saw the sunset from my back balcony, as I do most clinical days. I was too choked up to speak much during post-conference, so I called Dad that evening and told him I had seen two babies born that day. He immediately went into the story of when I was born; we laughed and cried together like we always do when he tells me that 5 pounds is so tiny that he could hold my head in his palm and the rest of me on his forearm. "But," he said, "they never get too big for you to hold in your heart even if they go off to nursing school and call you the first time they see the best miracle."

—Cheri N. Warren, BSN graduate, Texas

Getting and giving respect on the floor: your clinical instructors

The relationship between clinical instructors and nursing students is a unique one. You can end up spending 8 hours a day with your instructors, sometimes 3 or 4 days a week. You share breakfast, lunch, and sometimes dinner. You breathe the same air, touch the same patients, and keep the same schedule. Yet there is some tension because—even more than the instructors who teach objectively graded classes—clinical instructors have control over whether or not you pass the course.

" a student speaks

"I have had [both positive and negative] experiences with clinical instructors. My first instructor was easygoing and didn't push us at all. We needed to be pushed and forced to learn things, but she didn't do that. She didn't give us a lot of feedback, and she made it easy for us. My second semester was a complete change. My instructor was also my professor for my med-surg class, so she knew what we were learning and drilled us on it. She made sure we did our work each night, and she gave us hard and challenging assignments. It was a shock when I first had her, but I really appreciated her by the end. She worked just as hard as we did and made sure we knew our stuff."

— **Jessica Wheeler, BSN graduate, Connecticut**

Think of your clinical instructors as one of nursing school's most valuable resources. After all, your clinical instructor is something you want to be: a nurse. There is plenty of formal teaching that goes on in the clinical setting, but just as much happens over coffee, at breaks, and while waiting for post-conference to start. Ask your instructors about places where they've worked and patients they've taken care of. Even ask them why they became a nurse in the first place. Don't be afraid to ask, ask, ask. Clinical instructor positions are not known for being cushy jobs (I can't imagine supervising 10 students like me), so chances are that if your instructors are there, it's because they actually want to teach.

You have probably already noticed that each instructor has an individual style of teaching and areas of particular emphasis. I have heard nurse-educators refer to this as "faculty variability," whereas students might call it "personality quirks." Call it what you like, it pays to figure out what each instructor thinks is important so that you can avoid alarming them. For example, some instructors might like you to take full responsibility for your patient's care, alerting the instructor only in case of a problem. Others want to be updated every 30 seconds. ("Mr. X, I'm currently doing Patient Y's AM care. We've already completed the bath; I am going to get some lotion for her back now.") If you find out where your instructor is on this spectrum, you won't annoy them with excess detail or scare them by not giving enough.

Some students find that the most stressful times between students and instructors are the first day of a clinical rotation and the last. On the first day, the instructor is eyeing you up. He doesn't want you to mess up, hurt a patient or yourself—or his license, which is potentially in jeopardy as long as he is supervising you. If you convince him that you're prepared and safe, you'll both breathe easier.

On the last day of a clinical rotation, instructors are concerned that students may not have met all the clinical objectives. They don't want to wake up from a sound sleep a month after the rotation ends thinking, "Oh, no, Johnny Jones never demonstrated that he could flush a heparin lock." One easy way to avoid this situation is to review the clinical objectives for the course weekly (these should have been provided at orientation) and remind the instructor if you haven't had an opportunity to demonstrate your skills in some area. For more information on this topic, see *The process of learning procedures*.

The Process of Learning Procedures

It's a rare student nurse who doesn't recall with trepidation their first attempt at an IM injection. Many students find the process of learning how to perform nursing procedures challenging. It would be lovely to have the opportunity to watch a procedure done multiple times before attempting it. In the real world, however, students have to take advantage of the limited opportunities to practice procedures as they arise. Here are some students' suggestions about how to make the best of the opportunities that come your way.

- "Beg for the chance to do procedures. One way to be ahead of the pack is to read up on common procedures so that if the opportunity presents itself you can have the guts to say, 'I am prepared to do that.'"

- "Before you get your clinical instructors to come and observe you doing something, have everything ready so they don't have to wait for you. Once when I wanted to do a complicated dressing on a patient, my staff nurse pulled me into the supply room and started handing me supplies. When I showed up at my instructor's side with the policy and procedure manual read, supplies in hand, and a confident smile on my face, she was surprised but she let me do it."

(Continued)

The Process of Learning
Procedures (Continued)

- "Realize that even if you are completely prepared, you may get a surprise. For my first heparin injection, I waltzed confidently into the room, explained the procedure to the patient, and then proceeded to look for his umbilicus—which had been eliminated in his multiple abdominal surgeries. I looked for a few seconds and then turned around and mouthed to my instructor, 'He doesn't have an umbilicus.' She just nodded. I turned back around, estimated where the area around the umbilicus would have been, and gave the heparin there. I was grateful for my clinical instructor's calm handling of the situation."

- "Patients are so sick in hospitals these days that they are usually going to be focused on that and not on you and the fact that you are doing your first IM or whatever. Even if you are kind of nervous, you don't have to worry because while other nursing students and the staff might be able to tell that you're nervous, the patient probably won't."

- "Before explaining a procedure, ask the patient how much information they want about what you are doing. For example, one time when I was administering meds via a nasogastric tube, I was talking my patient through the procedure and I was very impressed with myself because I thought I was being so thorough. The patient finally blurted out, 'Good God, just get it over with, lady!' I was startled and embarrassed but (later) appreciated his honesty."

- "Don't be surprised if you are nervous. There was a Navy corpsman in my friend's class who had carried severed limbs from the battlefield but suddenly forgot how to change a Foley bag when someone was watching him. I guess he forgot temporarily that faking it is a time-honored nursing procedure. Who would feel competent to suction a tracheotomy the first time they do it?"

- "Make sure you've read up and practiced before you do any procedure. If the patient asks if you've ever done this before, I think it's important to be honest. You can say something like, 'I've been trained to do this.' And point out that your clinical instructor will be right there."

- "It helps you, the patient, and your instructor if you act really confident when you do any procedure for the first time."

- "Avoid excessive caffeine intake on clinical mornings. Too much caffeine will make your hands shake, especially when you're nervous, making it even harder to do procedures."

If a problem develops

" students speak

"Most [of my experiences with clinical instructors] were negative; most instructors were not supportive and were rude and dismissive to students. . . . We were quizzed on our [clinical paperwork] publicly and sometimes abusively."

— **Viane Frye, AD student, Florida.**

"To be honest, I never had a negative experience with a clinical instructor. I heard of people who did, but I never did. I always tried to be as well informed as I could be and even if I was unsure, I tried to adopt the 'never let 'em see you sweat' attitude. I always tried to listen to their advice, and I valued their knowledge. I never let myself feel intimidated. I think that's the first mistake people make. The most intimidating instructors are real people with real feelings; you shouldn't have any reason to let yourself be intimidated."

— **Jenny Smith, AD graduate, Oregon.**

Some instructors have the "I'll let you know if you do something wrong" approach and are then surprised when students run like mortified jackrabbits when they see the instructor coming. If you have one of these instructors, summon up your intestinal fortitude (as my grandmother would say) and request that you be given both positive *and* negative feedback.

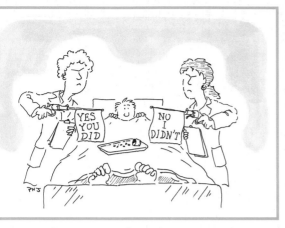

Sometimes communication breaks down between instructors and students and misunderstandings arise. This happens most often during hectic activity on the floor when you and your instructor are both trying to juggle the communication among patients, family, and staff in addition to the direct communication you are having with each other. If you find yourself confused by what the instructor is saying to you (either verbally or nonverbally), it may help to take the instructor aside and ask, "Mr./Ms./Dr. X (insert name of clinical instructor here), what is your expectation of me in this situation?" Your instructor may be surprised by your directness, but at least they'll see that you are trying to understand what they are conveying to you.

If you don't have an opportunity in the middle of a situation with a patient or family member, you can always ask a similar question after the dust clears, for example, "Do you feel I handled this situation appropriately, or should I have handled it in a different way?" Again, they may be surprised, but there is no way to know what they are thinking if you don't ask, and being proactive will save you both time.

If the problem persists

Of course, we've all heard stories of verbal abuse at the hands of clinical instructors. It's the "dirty little secret" of nursing school. Unfortunately, there are still old-school clinical instructors out there who confuse teaching with hazing. No doubt this was how they were taught and they believe—despite lots of research to the contrary—that somehow, if they make students anxious enough, they will learn more, or that they are doing students a service by "toughening them up." No matter what the motivation, this is what sociologists call "horizontal oppression" and nursing students call "a pain in the behind."

If you find yourself stuck with an instructor who is not treating you with respect, step back a bit and do a reality check with trustworthy classmates or a relatively objective third party. Describe the situation as carefully as you can and ask them if it sounds like there really is an ongoing problem or if you need to change your behavior or expectations.

If you are convinced that there is a problem, you have a few alternatives. The first option is that you can simply ignore the problem and hope that it goes away. Since clinical rotations are finite, this may be a viable option, especially if the situation is not interfering with your ability to learn and if the problem is rather mild. This may be your only choice if your classmates are unable or unwilling to back you up or if you know (based on past experiences or information from a reputable source) that student complaints are not usually taken seriously at your school. If you're going to take this route, find plenty of outside support, and get some sleep and work on your boundaries, because it may be a very long semester.

If you do want to confront the situation, discuss it with the instructor first. This is a professional courtesy and allows the instructor to share their view of the situations and interactions that have been causing your angst. Because nursing instructors are human, too, they occasionally act in ways that are less than ideal, especially under stressful circumstances. Perhaps their socks were too tight one day, or perhaps they were afraid for a patient's safety in a certain situation. They may have been taking care of a sick parent or dealing with an unruly toddler for 2 hours before they even hit the clinical floor. None of these situations excuse your instructor for being disrespectful to you, but if you know the instructor is struggling, perhaps you can work together to make the best of the situation for both of you.

When you chat with your instructor, try to make the exchange as nonconfrontational as possible. Use all those people skills nurses are so famous for, and make "I" statements (such as "I feel . . ." rather than "You make me feel . . .") so that your instructor will not feel accused. At the same time, be direct enough to get your point across. You don't want them scratching their head 2 hours later and wondering, "What was Matilda Metallica talking about anyway?"

If you aren't satisfied with the outcome of this discussion, there is assuredly an established procedure for dealing with complaints at your school. If you find out what that chain of command is and follow it, you'll have a better chance of resolving your complaint. And don't forget to document every contact you make during the process, in case you need to refer back to it later.

Even if you are delighted beyond words with your clinical experience, it is still important to maintain detailed records of your rotations. For example, each day after clinical, document what (in general) you did, the number of patients you took care of, and, most important, how you met the stated clinical objectives. Also, keep copies of any paperwork that you give to the instructor, along with paperwork that has been returned to you. This paperwork will be a good resource for further clinical rotations. In addition, because the clinical grade is most often a subjective one, this paperwork documents your work in case you have a conflict with an instructor about a grade.

Getting and giving respect on the floor: your classmates

Getting along

Not since "plays well with others" was part of the criteria for being promoted from kindergarten to first grade has teamwork been so important to your future. To succeed in your clinical rotations, communicate as often and as clearly as possible with your classmates. Classmates can be your best moral support. You'll find that it's mighty handy to have an extra pair of hands around when you put the thigh-high compression hose on your first knee-replacement patient who still has all of the staples in.

Don't ever randomly badmouth a classmate to a clinical instructor, no matter how annoying that classmate is. Speaking ill of your classmates is like making an announcement on the public address system: "Attention, all interested parties: I cannot work on a team."

Classmates and cultural competency

You've probably heard numerous lectures on cultural competency and even had to do a number of written projects or papers on cultural issues. However, cultural competency occasionally takes a bit of a battering in some circles when it is perceived as just another term that means "politically correct."

a student speaks

"I had one classmate who drove me absolutely out of my gourd at clinical. I don't know what her problem was, but she was condescending with African-American students. She assumed that every African-American student came from a drug-infested neighborhood. She would always ask me questions about gunshot wounds and about street names of drugs that patients might be using, which made no sense because I grew up in the suburbs and didn't know any more than she did. I sat her down and told her what I'd observed. She told me I was just being 'too sensitive.' I'm still glad I talked with her, because at least it's off my conscience. I wish she would have listened a bit more closely when our instructors covered cultural competency!"
— **M.L, BSN student, Iowa**

This is a fallacy, however. Cultural competency is not about saying the right magic words to avoid offending anyone. Cultural competency is learning about people who may be from a very different social, racial, ethnic, or economic background from us so that we can treat them with respect, whether they are classmates, instructors, or patients.

A large part of learning cultural competency is recognizing the stereotypes that we hold about groups of people. For example, in the above scenario you can see how the condescending nursing student was reacting to a stereotype she had of African-Americans. Some stereotypes are more malicious than others, but they are all harmful in that they create barriers between people. These barriers are detrimental both to working effectively as a patient-care team and to providing responsible care. See the Resources section at the end of this chapter for some good Web sites relevant to these issues.

Getting and giving respect on the floor: your patients

Confidentiality

" a student speaks

"I tried to always be extra careful about patient confidentiality because our instructors emphasize it so much, but I didn't really have any personal feelings about it until after my first year of nursing school. The summer between my first and second years of school, I had to have surgery and ended up in a hospital in the very small town where I live. I knew many of the nurses because they were all friends of my family or parents of my children's classmates. Everyone was very careful about my personal information except for one nurse who worked the night shift. About 3 days after I was discharged, I ran into her at the grocery store. She made an indiscreet comment that gave away the nature of my hospitalization to my 8-year-old, who was with me. We had explained to him in general terms why I had had to have surgery but were not going to be specific until we knew about the final lab results. As it was, I was fine, but my son was caused a lot of needless worry because of one person's lack of discretion. Now my friends call me the confidentiality tyrant because I am always making sure charts are not left open, paperwork is not left sitting around, etc. And I never, never, never talk with a patient about their diagnosis or condition in front of family members unless I talk with the patient about it alone and get the okay first."

— S.L., BSN student, Alaska

In a busy teaching hospital, it is a constant challenge to keep patients' personal information personal. Students want to see and learn; that's why we're at the hospital in the first place. Patients, however, are at the hospital because they are sick or injured and are very vulnerable. It is essential to remain constantly aware of our patients' vulnerability and their rights as human beings so that we do not inadvertently compromise either their privacy or their confidentiality.

There are a number of ways in which student nurses can contribute to a hospital environment that makes patient confidentiality a top priority. First, refuse to carry on conversations about a patient within earshot of other patients or visitors. This may require some assertiveness on your part when, for example, your primary nurse approaches you in the hallway when you come back from lunch break and attempts to give you an impromptu report about your patient. I'm not suggesting that the only appropriate action is to bolt away from the nurse, screaming as you run down the hallway, "DOESN'T ANYONE HERE CARE ABOUT CONFIDENTIALITY???!!!" Instead, you can suggest that the two of you step into a nearby empty room or a corner of the nurses' station to continue the conversation.

Second, zealously guard your patient's paperwork. Don't leave charts sitting open, even at the nurses' station, and always double-check to make sure you have not left your notes from report or patient printouts when you exit a room. On any piece of patient information that leaves the hospital (for example, if you get a printout to prepare for clinical), black out the patient's name and replace it with their initials. Do the same for any piece of paper that you're going to submit to your instructor, unless you are given very explicit instructions to the contrary.

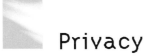

Privacy

Maintaining patients' personal privacy is another challenge that nursing students face. It's natural—and common—to get embarrassed the first few times we perform intimate care. L.L., a BSN student from Massachusetts, said, "The first time I had to help someone on the toilet, I thought I literally was going to die of embarrassment. The patient was a male, and about my age. I knew I was blushing, but I couldn't do anything about it. Finally, the patient said, 'Relax, honey, you're just doing your job.' I was able to relax, and we got the whole ordeal completed with no problems. After that I started reminding myself that I could have a matter-of-fact attitude about personal care while still being compassionate."

In addition to being matter of fact about patient care, it is important to make sure patients are modestly covered when performing any procedure. Also, always ask—and wait for—an answer before you touch a conscious patient, even to take a blood pressure. For more hints on meeting the psychosocial needs of nonresponsive patients, see *Patients in a coma CAN hear you*. The writer spent time in a coma due to kidney failure, recovered, and is now a second-year nursing student.

Patients in a Coma CAN Hear You: Hints on Meeting the Psychosocial Needs of Nonresponsive Patients

My experience with unresponsiveness comes firsthand. In July 1994 I was in a coma for 5 days after my kidneys shut down. This is a brief account of what I experienced while I was in that coma.

First of all, you should know that the patient is not really in any pain if they are well medicated, but they can still hear you and, in a way, respond to you. When I was comatose, I can tell you that I felt like I was either standing or sitting by my bed most of the time. Now, I don't know if that was due to the medication, but after I came out of the coma, it made me feel better to know I was still "there" even when I was still in the coma.

Do not let anyone tell you that a patient in a coma cannot hear you! I can very clearly remember my dad reading fly fishing magazines to me when I was in the coma. And I also heard my mom and my nephrologist telling me everything that was happening. When they came in and started talking, they said my heart rate rose. They asked me about it afterwards, and I told them that I would get very angry with them because I was trying to talk to them when they were talking to me! They just couldn't hear me.

Definitely ask your patient's family if there is a certain song the patient likes, or a certain spot on their body they like rubbed. My mom knew that I liked my hair and head rubbed, and while I was in the coma, she would rub my head. This would slow my respirations and heart rate. If you know of anything you think a patient will respond to, try it!

If I could tell anyone just one thing about a loved one being in a coma, it would be to talk to them as much as possible. They are still there and can hear you.

—Darrell Fretwell, AD student, Mesa Community College, Mesa, Arizona

Not for the Weak of Stomach

Here are some students' suggestions for dealing with the unpleasant smells and sights of nursing.

- "Use a little bit of menthol cold stuff right inside your nose. It will cover up bad smells because all you'll be smelling is menthol."

- "Before you go in to do a dressing, ask the primary nurse what the wound looks like. It's better than being surprised when you take off the old dressing."

- "If you are cleaning up a patient and feel like you're about to gag, force yourself to cough. It seems nearly impossible to cough and gag at the same time. This will save both you and the patient embarrassment, especially since once you start gagging, it's hard to stop."

- "Right before you do a particularly difficult dressing or colostomy care, pop a piece of very strongly flavored gum in your mouth. I've found that cinnamon works best."

Sometimes personal care can be difficult in a different way, especially if you have the unfortunate curse of a being squeamish. Don't despair—dealing with things that either smell or look unpleasant is an acquired nursing art; for tips see *Not for the weak of stomach.*

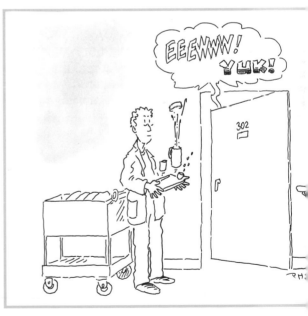

Getting and giving respect on the floor: the staff

You can learn a great deal from the staff nurses, not only about how to perform various procedures but also about how to talk with people, how to listen, and how to work bathroom breaks into a busy schedule.

Most nursing students I talked with said the best way to develop a good relationship with a primary nurse in particular and the hospital staff in general is to take the initiative and be eager to do the work. Depending on how far along you are in your nursing school journey, this can mean making sure your patients get AM care, ambulated, fed, and given meds on time and without being told.

Nurses may deal with different-level students from different schools every day of the week, so instead of assuming that they know what you can and can't do, bring the subject up when you get report. Also, if you aren't on the floor for the entire shift, let your primary nurse know at the beginning of the shift and remind them again when it's close to your time to leave.

I think it's important to remember that floor nurses are not paid to teach nursing students. As our first semester clinical instructor reminded us, it's the institution that contracts to take students, not the individual nurses. Of course, that doesn't mean that there should be open season on nursing students as soon as they step on the floor or that staff nurses have no obligation to cooperate with nursing students. In most hospitals, however, staff nurses are extremely busy and fairly stressed out, so any additional responsibilities may seem burdensome. My general experience has been that the more students can be self-directed, helpful, and low-maintenance, the more time a primary nurse will be able and willing to spend with them.

This is definitely a balancing act, though. The days are gone (we hope) when nursing students are serfs to be used and abused as free labor. The purpose of clinical rotations is to learn, not to see how many bedpans you can scrub out in 8 hours. It may be helpful to think of the energy and effort that you bring to the task as barter for the extra time that the staff must take to communicate with you and teach you.

When you don't like what you see

The one thing I wish I'd known before I started clinical rotations is that hospital nursing is in a state of crisis. Don't ask me how I missed this. All my friends who were in nursing worked in the community, and although they certainly struggled, they all seemed happy to call nursing their profession. I was shocked when I got onto the hospital floor and encountered extremely overworked and stressed-out nurses, some of whom seemed very intent on discouraging future nurses from their career path. For example, in my first semester, a classmate and I accompanied another classmate, who was pregnant and experiencing severe dizziness, to the emergency room. When the triage nurse found out our major, he spent 10 minutes urging us to "get out now while you still can," until my ill friend spoke up. "Could you please," she asked meekly, with her head buried in her hands to quell her dizziness, "save the lecture until after you've at least taken my vital signs?"

I really believe this nurse's intention was to save us the pain and difficulty that he was dealing with. The crisis in health care has created a crisis in nursing, and many good, strong, competent nurses are leaving the profession or becoming burnt out. This does not mean that nursing students should find another major, only that students should be aware of the challenges of nursing in the current health-care environment and should be actively advocating for change in the system. These issues of advocacy and the health-care crisis are explored fully in Chapter 9.

ROLL IN THE ROLE MODELS

Because of this crisis and the burnout it has caused, it is important for student nurses not to expect that nurses on the floor where they do clinical rotations will necessarily be good choices for role models. Many floor nurses at clinical sites have a lot to offer nursing students and are very willing to share their enthusiasm and expertise. However, when this happens, students should consider this an extra bonus. Students should actively seek out encouragement and mentoring from other sources. More information on finding and working with a mentor can be found in Chapter 10.

RESOURCES

Web sites

ASK DR. WEIL

www.askdrweil.com

Dr. Andrew Weil is a Harvard-educated author and physician who is well known for his teachings about nontraditional medicine. At this Web site, he gets 500 questions a week and his staff pick out five for him to answer. At last count, more than 600 questions were archived. I've included this site here because, even if you haven't visited it, one of your patients will have.

BLACK HEALTH NET

www.blackhealthnet.com

This site contains articles, a history of African-American medicine, a question-and-answer section, a discussion forum, and related links. You can also search from here for information on the rest of the Internet about the health of African-Americans.

ETHNIC COMMUNITY HEALTH PROFILES

www.health.qld.gov.au/hssb/cultdiv/home.htm

Brought to you by the energetic folks at the Queensland (Australia) Health Information Network, this site is neatly divided into three sections: Cultural Diversity, Guidelines to Practice, and Checklists for Cultural Assessment. If you need to know about death and dying, diet and food, or gender and modesty practices of a certain cultural group, this is the place to visit. It also addresses challenges when working with special populations such as children and youth, women, and victims of torture and trauma.

ETHNOMED

www.hslib.washington.edu/clinical/ethnomed/index.html

This site is a collection of health profiles from the University of Washington. It includes Ethiopian, Somalian, Eritrean, Cambodian, and Vietnamese cultural groups.

KIDS' HEALTH-LAB TEST EXPLANATION FOR KIDS

http://www.kidshealth.org.parent/system/

This page is meant to help parents understand and explain lab tests to their children, but it's a valuable resource for beginning nursing students because it's so nontechnical. The quick downloading time is an added bonus.

MEDICAL CHOICE'S PHOTO ROUNDS

www.mdchoice.com/photo/phototoc.asp

If you're easily grossed out and the *Not for the weak of stomach* tips in this chapter didn't help you, you can build your tolerance slowly by spending a few minutes a day at this site. There are pictures of everything from a child with varicella to an individual with two amputated legs from a train wreck. Not suggested lunchtime surfing material.

MEDI-SMART FORUM

http://medi-smart.com/proc.html

This site contains numerous assessment tips and tools.

MENTAL HEALTH NET

www.mentalhelp.net/selfhelp

If you have a patient with a mental health problem who is able to get online and is seeking support, this is the first place to send them. It's searchable by geographic location and by disorder.

MULTICULTURAL HEALTH LINKS

http://www.lib.iun.indiana.edu/trannurs.htm

This Web site provides many transcultural and multicultural health links, including ones to ethnic groups, religious groups, and other special populations.

NATIONAL CENTER FOR COMPLEMENTARY AND ALTERNATIVE MEDICINE (NCCAM)

http://nccam.nih.gov/

This federal government Web site includes research, training, and information for both practitioners and consumers on complementary and alternative medicine.

RESPIRATORY THERAPY CENTER

www.rtcorner.com

Having trouble with breath sounds? Get on a speaker-equipped computer and head right to this page.

RX LIST

www.rxlist.com

This is the best drug information site on the Internet, in my opinion. It contains a comprehensive list of meds that you can search not just by generic and chemical names but also by parts of names (useful if the patient can only tell you "Well, I take a blue pill, and it begins with an N and ends in a vowel"). It also shows interactions with herbal and other over-the-counter drugs, which is information difficult to find elsewhere. You can even search for a medication by the imprint code found on the pill or capsule. Thanks to links to an abbreviated form of Taber's Medical Dictionary, you can look up definitions of nearly any word on the site with a single click. Extremely useful.

WOUND CARE NET

www.woundcarenet.com

All you ever wanted to know about wound care, and possibly a lot less. Again, not lunchtime surfing material.

Yes, You Can Avoid: Anxiety, Severe, Related to the Upcoming NCLEX

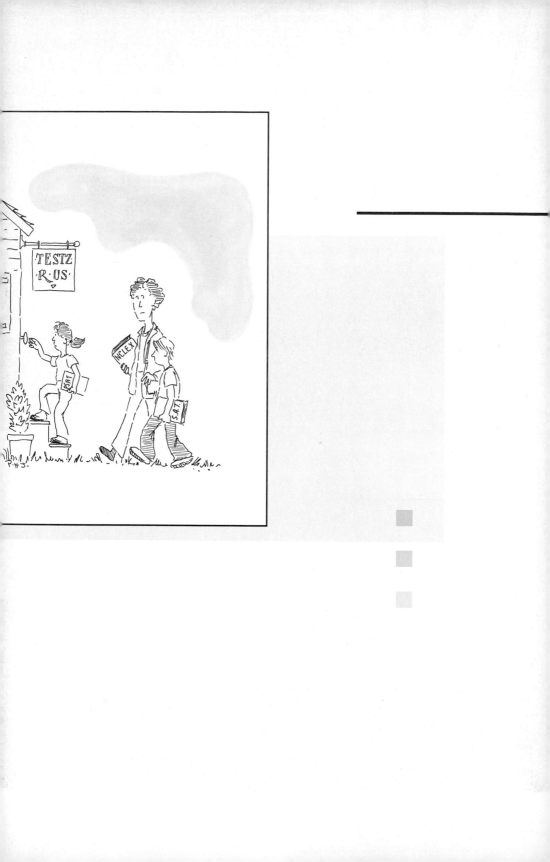

CHAPTER 8

Yes, You Can Avoid: Anxiety, Severe, Related to the Upcoming NCLEX

" a student speaks

"When the final exam was over, a bunch of us went out to celebrate. We went to a restaurant close to school and got a table. We sat down and looked at each other. No one had anything to say. It was like at the end of [the movie] *Poseidon Adventure*. Okay, we were among the survivors. Now what?"

— C.T., AD graduate, New Jersey

It's hard to believe. Graduation has come and gone, you've been pinned, you've toasted your success, and you've written thank-you notes for all the great graduation gifts you've received. You are becoming reacquainted with family members and roommates estranged by the rigors of nursing school. You've burned your clinical uniform in a grand celebratory ritual.

Don't be surprised if you find yourself feeling lost, wandering aimlessly around the house and seriously contemplating writing a care plan for your cat. Many new grads experience an emotional letdown after graduating. Think about it—you've spent at least 2 and possibly up to 5 years of eating, drinking, and sleeping nursing school. Like it or not, nursing school has taken over a great deal of your time, energy, and money. It's great to have that time and energy back, and when you get your first job as a nurse, you'll start to recover some of the money. Still, it's natural to feel a sense of loss. In addition, you have been under stress since the day you first sat down in Nursing 101. You have had to shut off some of the stress response to reach your goal, but now you may feel wrung out after such a long time in the throes of a "fight-or-flight" response. It's okay. Take a deep breath and repeat after me: "I finished nursing school. I can do anything, including taking the NCLEX."

Anticipation

Planning

Now that you're out of school, don't forget to keep in touch with your classmates during the transitional period. In the olden days, the NCLEX, also known as the state boards, was offered only twice a year. All the new grads would pile into an auditorium as large as a football field and take the test, which took the better part of 2 days. Since 1994, however, the NCLEX has been given in a computerized format that new grads usually take at a testing center near their home, on a date and at a time selected by each individual. While this no doubt eliminates some of the more stressful aspects of taking the NCLEX, new grads no longer have the solidarity that results from automatically having a test date that's the same as their classmates'. That's why it's important not to cut yourself off from your nursing school pals at this time. Plan times to get together and talk through NCLEX strategies, exchange job search leads, and generally hang out.

Registering

It's essential to understand who the different players are in the NCLEX registration game. The National Council of State Boards of Nursing (hereafter the NCSBN) is the group that develops the exam (as well as sells test prep materials) and that ultimately rules on any disputes about the way the test is administered. The Chauncey Group registers graduates to take the exam (unless you live in Illinois or Massachusetts, where there is a slightly different procedure) and sends you the Authorization to Test (hereafter known as the ATT). If you lose your ATT, or need to make changes to your ATT (for example, if your name is spelled wrong), you contact the Chauncey Group. Sylvan Learning Centers, Inc., is the nationwide entity that administers the exam, so you'll go to a local Sylvan Learning Center to take the NCLEX. Your state board of nursing issues your license and makes some decisions about how the exam is administered in your state.

The procedure for licensing varies slightly from state to state, but the general process is similar everywhere. In order to understand this process, it's important to clearly understand that you are registering for two different but closely related things. You are applying for licensure as a registered nurse and you are applying to take the NCLEX, the exam that allows you to obtain your license.

The first step in the process is finishing your classes and taking your final exams. When your instructors have submitted your grades to the school, your school should provide you with an application for licensure from your state board of nursing, as well as an application for graduate nurse (GN) status if it is available in your state. The school should also give you something called the *NCLEX Examination Candidate Bulletin,* which is issued by the NCSBN and provides detailed information about registering for the NCLEX. You also need to obtain something called the education program code. This five-digit code is unique to your school of nursing. It should be given to you at the same time as your *NCSBN Examination Candidate Bulletin,* since you need it to complete your registration for the NCLEX.

Submit your application for licensure to your state's board of nursing. Submit your application to take the NCLEX to the Chauncey Group, unless you live in Massachusetts or Illinois, where you submit it directly to the NCSBN. If you register by mail to take the NCLEX, you must send a certified check or money order for $120 and (this is the tricky part) you make it out to the NCSBN, although you send it to the Chauncey Group. You can't use a credit card if you register by mail. However, you can register with your credit card on the phone. This process is quicker, but they tack on a $9.25 "service charge," so you'll pay a total of $129.95.

After you've submitted your application for licensure and your application to take the NCLEX, you have plenty of time to develop stress-related hypertension while you wait for the Chauncey Group to send your ATT. The moment you receive your ATT, you can call the Sylvan Learning Center nearest you to get a date to take the test. A list of centers is included with your ATT. If you are taking the exam for the first time, you will need to propose a date for taking the NCLEX that is within 30 days of your call.

Picking a time and place

It is to your advantage to complete this initial paperwork process as soon as possible, even if you think you may want to delay taking the test for some reason. The earlier you get your paperwork done, the better the chances of being able to get your first preference for time and place at Sylvan. This may be critical if you live in an area where there are a several schools of nursing and many graduates are competing for available time slots at the testing centers.

You can go to any testing center in your state to take the test. If you have trouble getting a timely date in your area, you may want to call around to other testing centers in your region of the state to see if they can accommodate you earlier. However, traveling will only increase the stressfulness of taking the exam, so avoid this situation if you can by getting your paperwork in early.

Be aware that once you get your ATT, you don't have an unlimited amount of time to schedule the test. Your ATT is valid only for a period set by your state's board of nursing. This can be from 55 to 999 days from the date your ATT is issued, depending on your state. If you don't take your test between those dates, you have to start the registration process for the test all over and (groan) pay the fees again.

Plan to take the test as soon as you can reasonably be ready. If you have a job waiting for you or you need your license by a certain date, your decision about when to take the NCLEX will be made for you. Otherwise, plan for a date that will allow you to complete your individualized study plan (see next section) with at least a week to spare. Depending on your schedule and the amount of reviewing you think you need, this might be as little as 3 weeks or as much as

3 months from the time you start studying. Most students and educators I've talked to advise against waiting more than 4 months to take the exam, no matter what the circumstances.

One advantage of taking the NCLEX at community-based testing centers is that you can pick a time of day when you are most (as my grandma says) bright-eyed and bushy-tailed. Testing centers schedule 5-hour blocks of time for the test, and most close no later than 10 PM. This means that you can usually pick a time between 8 AM and 5 PM to start the test. If you have to accept a time of day that is not ideal for you in order to take the NCLEX in a timely fashion, don't despair. You took nursing tests at your school's whim, not yours, and were still able to get through; you can do the same on the NCLEX.

Finally, when you call to schedule the date and time, write it down. There's even a handy little spot on your ATT to do just that. Sylvan doesn't send out any type of confirmation, so whatever notation you make will be the only reminder you have.

The NCLEX in a nutshell

The NCLEX is made up of multiple-choice questions much like you had all through nursing school. However, since April 1994, the NCLEX has been administered via computer instead of paper and pencil. This test is of a type called, quite aptly, computerized adaptive testing because everyone who takes the NCLEX gets a test that is custom-made for them.

This is how the NCLEX works: Suzy Skillful goes into the testing center, registers, and shows the helpful, attentive attendant at the front desk her ATT and two pieces of identification. Suzy is fingerprinted and photographed for identification purposes. She then signs some paperwork and is given scrap paper and a pencil, which she must return to the desk monitor when she leaves (the only souvenir of the NCLEX will

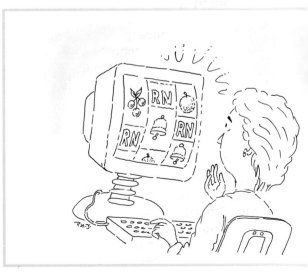

be her license). Suzy is escorted to a smallish study carrel, where she sits down on what may or may not be a noncreaky chair and faces the computer. After taking a short tutorial on how to use the computer and answering three sample questions, she starts answering questions that really count. The computer displays a question, which Suzy answers by selecting the correct item with the space bar and hitting the ENTER key. If she gets the question right, the computer gives her a slightly harder question. If she gets the question wrong, the computer gives her a slightly easier question. Suzy can't go back and change any of her answers once she has hit the ENTER key for that particular question, and she can't skip a question. This dance continues, with the computer providing questions and Suzy answering them and the computer deciding what question to display next until it can determine Suzy's skill level. She'll answer between 75 and 265 questions. When the computer shuts off, it will know whether Suzy passed. However, this is not information the computer is going to share with Suzy. She will have to wait for about 4 weeks and follow her state board of nursing's procedure for finding out the results.

Preparation

Assessing your needs

" a student speaks

"I spent too much time studying pharmacology and not enough time studying med-surg basics. I wasted a lot of time studying for the NCLEX because I didn't know what my strengths and weaknesses were."

— F.P., BSN graduate, New Jersey

When your school offers the National League for Nursing (NLN) pre-assessment test, take it, even if it is optional. (Some schools require a certain score on the NLN test to graduate). Regardless of your score, taking this exam will alert you to content areas that may need special attention in your review plan.

If the NLN's pre-assessment test is not available, you will need to use some other tool to pinpoint your areas of strength and weakness. For example, you can take one of the sample tests available in NCLEX review books. Note which content areas you had difficulty with and which type of questions you typically missed. If something seems amiss about the results (for example, you did poorly on questions about infectious diseases and you had a PhD in microbiology before you went to nursing school), take another test, ideally from a different book. Compare the results and see what kind of pattern develops.

Mapping out a study plan

Once you have an idea of your current NCLEX-taking skill level, you are ready to come up with a study plan. The first part of your studying should consist of an overall content review, concentrating on content areas in which you are weak. You can do this by using commercially available prep materials, taking an NCLEX prep class, or reviewing class notes. Remember that NCLEX review really is supposed to be a review. If you try to relearn every random detail you learned about tuberculosis or asthma or arthrogryposis throughout your nursing school career, you will make yourself and everyone around you utterly miserable. Concentrate on the most important information in each content area and note how the pieces of each part of your nursing knowledge fit together to make a whole.

After you complete your content review, you should spend a significant period of time answering (and then reviewing) NCLEX-type questions from review books. Many students told me they answered as many as 6000 questions during their NCLEX preparation. Doing test questions helps you become familiar with the structure of different types of questions, develop a rhythm, and become more adept at analyzing test questions for clues about how to pick out the right answer from the other answers that serve as distractors. As you work your way through the questions, review the rationale for each answer and make sure you understand not only why certain answers were wrong, but also why the correct answer was the most correct. If you work through questions this way, you not only practice question-answering skills, but also get in extra content review as well.

Answering an incredible number of questions can have the additional benefit of increasing your test-taking confidence. The more questions you answer, the less the likelihood that the computer will be able to throw you a question that has a structure you have not seen before. I had completed 6500 questions by the time I took the NCLEX. I'm not sure how useful the last 4500 questions were. I am sure I was very sick of looking at NCLEX questions. However, by the time I sat down at the computer, I felt completely ready to take the test. There were things about the test that surprised me (mostly how many questions I was asked about borderline personality disorder), but my feeling of readiness helped me not to panic when I received a question that I thought I might not know. Most students I talked with completed 2000 to 4000 practice questions.

If you have consistently struggled with test taking, you may need more than practice questions to develop your skills. It might be wise to invest in either a private NCLEX tutor or a commercial test-preparation course that includes test-taking skills as well as content review.

To develop your individualized study plan, first calculate how long you intend to spend doing content review. If you are going to take a test-preparation course to review content, you can look at the number of hours that the course runs and add in any additional time that the course developers suggest for study to come up with a ballpark figure. If you are doing content review on your own, calculating your time can be a bit trickier. You may need to study one section of content to see how long it takes you and then multiply that time by the number of content sections.

Second, spend a few hours doing practice questions and calculate the average number of questions you can do in an hour. Divide this figure by the number of questions you intend to complete to find out how many hours you should reserve for answering practice questions. Add the hours you need to spend on content review and the hours you need to spend on practice questions and—presto—you have the number of hours of review time that stand between you and the NCLEX. Don't spend too much time dwelling on this number though, or you may develop severe situational depression. Instead, get out your Dayplanner or personal digital assistant or whatever other tool you use for keeping track of your schedule and plot out blocks of time for NCLEX preparation. Keep in mind limitations that your child-care and work schedule may impose. Also, be mindful of how much time each day you can realistically hope to concentrate without your eyeballs bugging out of your head and your brain turning to overcooked pasta. Once you have your times plotted out and have added a week's padding to account for emergencies, you have your target NCLEX date.

The process I've described here is decidedly not rocket science, but developing a study plan for the NCLEX is vital because your plan can keep you on track and prevent you from overstudying. Do not let the NCLEX take over your life. If you use your study plan, you will be freed up to think about the NCLEX when you're reviewing for it and to think about other things when you're not. Perhaps you will still find yourself randomly seized with the thought "Myasthenia gravis! I've forgotten everything I ever knew about myasthenia gravis!" as you drive down the road or put away groceries. However, with a good study plan you can gently redirect your attention to the right turn you were making or to rearranging the freezer to accommodate the 5-gallon container of ice cream. "There is a time to worry about myasthenia gravis and a time to worry about right turns and ice cream" you will remind yourself, and continue on with your life.

Choosing review tools and options

There is an incredible amount of money to be made in the NCLEX preparation game, and so there is an unbelievable array of options for study helps. Just as you are budgeting time to study, budget money for test-prep materials, and then do not let the NCLEX take over your budget. For more information about selecting NCLEX preparation tools, see *Choosing multimedia review tools for NCLEX preparation, Choosing a review course,* and *Thoughts on choosing NCLEX review books.*

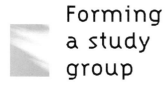

Forming a study group

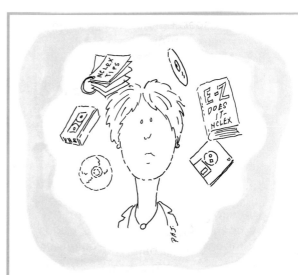

If you live in an area where there are several nursing schools, I suggest forming a study group with new graduates from other schools. Ideally,

Choosing Multimedia Tools
for NCLEX Preparation

Multimedia tools, such as cassette tapes, computer diskettes, and compact discs (CDs), can be quite useful in helping you prepare for the NCLEX. Keep these tips in mind when selecting these tools:

- CDs and 3.5-inch diskettes containing practice questions should mimic actual test conditions as closely as possible. This means they should use only the space bar and ENTER key for navigation and should randomize questions.

- If you buy books that come with a CD or diskette, make sure the practice questions on these electronic media are not in the book as well. When you take practice tests on the computer, you should be dealing with questions you have never seen before.

- Companies that produce NCLEX review courses often have audiocassette or video recordings of review courses for sale. These can be a useful alternative if you can't fit a review course into your schedule. However, ask if you can try before you buy. If the class was recorded using inferior equipment or if the instructor did not take into account the fact that the class was being taped (e.g., was unaware of the location of the recording equipment or wrote important information on the board), the tapes may not be useful.

- Online review options are burgeoning and have the benefits of being available 24 hours a day and instantly updateable. However, online courses and practice tests are usually quite expensive and can be time consuming if you are unfamiliar with the technology. Since most sites offer some type of free trial, you can easily compare the different features and price plans available and make an informed purchase.

these should be students from another type of program, for example, students from an AD program if you graduated from a BSN program, BSN students if you graduated from AD program. Each program will have had individual differences and areas of emphasis. Not only will you have the benefit of exposure to these individual differences and areas of emphasis, but you will also acquire valuable job-search allies and extend your professional network.

You can find students from other schools through Internet contacts, by posting notices on other campuses, and by calling or e-mailing members of the faculty of neighboring schools of nursing. Make sure to do this well before final exams or there may be no one around to read the e-mail or the notices.

Choosing a Review Course

Some schools require students to take an NCLEX review course as part of the academic requirements of the last semester and include the price of the class with the fees for that semester. Some students find these classes to be helpful, but others find them a waste of time. If you need help structuring your content review or could use some additional coaching on test-taking strategies, you will probably want to take a review course. The quality of review courses varies widely, so make sure you ask plenty of questions before you give up your hard-earned cash. Things to consider when choosing a course include the following:

- Does the review course incorporate some kind of diagnosis and assessment of students' test readiness at the beginning of the course?

- Does the course review content, test-taking strategies, or both?

- Who teaches the class? Nurses? Graduate students? Faculty members from a local school of nursing? Are the faculty members clinically current? How familiar are they with the specifics of NCLEX preparation?

- Ask to sit in on a class. Does the instructor encourage questions while still keeping the class focused and on track? Does the instructor seem knowledgeable, organized, and well prepared?

- How many students are in a typical class? What is the maximum number of students in a class?

- Does the class include any "take-away" information such as handouts or books?

- What kind of guarantee does the class offer? Are partial refunds available if a student is dissatisfied with the class and does not want to complete it?

- How often is the class offered?

- Does the course fee include any use of computer tutorials or other prep tools outside of class time?

Thoughts on Choosing
NCLEX Review Books

- A quick search of Amazon.com turns up more than 150 different books claiming to be useful to students preparing for the NCLEX. To help you make the right choice, ask your classmates, instructors, and study partners about the books they recommend. Many large online book distributors provide space for customers to write reviews of books they've bought. These reviews can be a valuable source of information.

- Since the quality of NCLEX books varies widely, do not buy any NCLEX review book without seeing it. If you want to order your books online, page through your choices at a local bookstore first.

- Look at content and features of books more than cost, since most NCLEX review books are priced competitively.

- Before buying a NCLEX review book, check to see if the format will be easy for you to use. For example, it is helpful to have questions on one side of the page and answers and rationales on the other side, rather than having the answers and rationales at the back of the book. Otherwise, you may spend half your NCLEX review time flipping pages. You can cover the answers with a piece of paper if you're tempted to peek.

- Some books contain both content review and sample questions. If you are getting your content review elsewhere (e.g., through a review course) and are only looking for practice questions, skip the book that has content so you can get more questions for your NCLEX review dollar.

- If you are looking for a book with content review, remember that the book with more pages is not necessarily the better choice. You are looking for content summary, not a record of every bit of information ever taught in any nursing school since the beginning of time.

- Many of the same companies that publish NCLEX review books also sell decks of NCLEX review cards. These cards can be good for reviewing content on the go but are less practical for completing practice questions. Ideally, at least part of your review should be done under actual test conditions, and looking over cards at the bus stop does not qualify.

Taking the test

Final preparation

Sometime in the last week before you take the test, do a test run to the Sylvan Learning Center at the same time of day you will be taking the test. This will allow you to double-check that your directions are accurate and note any glitches with public transportation or parking. Check for a coffee shop or restaurant near the testing center where you can sit and drink a cup of whatever liquid stimulates your brain in case you should arrive obscenely early on test day. Try different combinations of potential pretest foods to see which ones power up your thought processes most effectively.

Finally, inasmuch as you have control over the people, places, and things that annoy you, avoid them. If someone from church gets on your nerves, stay away from that person. Don't read the newspaper or open direct-mail solicitation ads. There is a time to worry about the state of the world, but the last few days before you take the NCLEX is not it.

If you smoke, practice going for 5 hours without a cigarette. Your lungs will be happy, and you will be less likely to be distracted by nicotine craving should you require all 5 hours to take the test. Review the visualization exercises in Chapter 2 and deep-breathing exercises in Chapter 5 of this book and practice them until they become second nature, especially if you are particularly anxious when you take tests.

No matter how unprepared you feel, stop studying at least 36 hours before you're scheduled to take the NCLEX. Use this time to do something relaxing and fun that will occupy your thoughts and keep them from straying to the test.

On the day of the test, leave sufficiently early that even a tidal wave, earthquake, and Godzilla on the loose combined would not keep you from getting to the testing center on time. If you arrive at the testing center 30 minutes early or less, check in with the front desk staff because they might let you take your exam early. Otherwise, wait in the coffee shop you found earlier so that you don't have to be exposed to everyone's else pretest jitters. It's easy enough to be anxious on one's own, without the help of strangers.

Handling the computer

By the time you sit down on your day of reckoning at the Sylvan Learning Center, you should have practiced enough with disks or CD-ROMs that use exactly the same keystrokes as the actual test that the computer is the least of your worries. However, should you become confused, remember that you can ask for help with the computer at any time, even after the test begins.

To review: You have to use only two keys to take the NCLEX—the space bar and the ENTER key. You use the space bar to move the cursor around the answer choices. You can tell when the space bar is indicating a particular answer because that answer will be highlighted. Once the space bar is highlighting the answer you want to pick, you actually have to hit the ENTER key twice before an answer is saved and you are thrown the next question.

Handling your anxiety

First, it is perfectly reasonable to be slightly anxious about taking the NCLEX. You have expended plenty of blood, sweat, and tears to come to this point. As one diploma grad told me, "I was in debt up to my ears and running out of money fast when I took the NCLEX. Passing was literally my meal ticket." Even if you're not in such dire financial straits, it's no small thing to be tested on years of accumulated knowledge. You would have to be comatose not to feel butterflies in your stomach at this point. Do not be anxious about being anxious.

Since you can't go back and change answers, treat each question as an exam in itself; once you hit the ENTER key the second time, immediately turn your attention to the next question. Tell yourself not to be surprised by anything. You are at a psychological disadvantage if you expect the computer to turn off at a certain number and it doesn't. So, if you can, avoid looking at the question number as you answer each question.

If you are distracted by the clicking of other people's computers or other such annoying sounds, you can ask for earplugs. Sylvan provides them, and they're disposable and not entirely unattractive.

Remember that rest breaks are built into the exam time. The computer forces you to take a 10-minute break after you've been sitting at the computer for 2 hours. After another hour and a half, you can take another break, but the computer does not enforce this one. The whole testing time is 5 hours, including the breaks and the computer tutorial. Use the breaks to rest your eyes (sleeping is not recommended) and do some deep breathing.

Finally, there are going to be other people close to you or next to you who may sit down at the computer as the same time as you do. They may get up before you, but ignore them! Sylvan administers many different tests, so you can realistically tell yourself that the person next to you who finished in 45 minutes wasn't even taking the NCLEX. Even if they were taking the NCLEX, you don't need to think about it. A little denial in this situation can go a long way.

Getting your results

The 3 to 4 weeks that it will take for your state board of nursing to send you either a license or a notification of failure will seem like an eternity. Some states participate in a 900-number system that enables you to get your results sooner, while others post results online. Hang in there and remind yourself that it's almost over.

If you don't pass

" a student speaks

"I didn't pass the NCLEX on the first try simply because I was so anxious. I was determined not to let it happen again. I took a Kaplan course and did everything they said to do. I went to every class, practiced the suggested amount of time on the computer, and used all their test-taking hints. I passed the second time around; in fact, the computer shut off after 75 questions. I've been working as an ER nurse for 4 years now, and no one at my job knows or cares that it took me two tries to pass the NCLEX."

— P. P., BSN graduate, Iowa

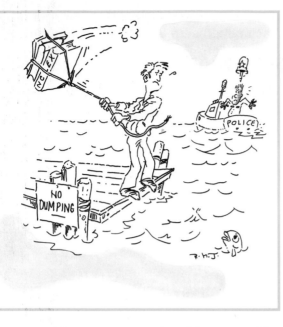

If you should fail the NCLEX on the first try, do not panic and do not let anyone tell you that this means you cannot be a nurse or that you will not be a good nurse. Failing the NCLEX means you failed the NCLEX. That's it.

While you wait for the 90 days to pass until you can retake your boards, review all your options. I suggest taking your results to your academic adviser from school or to an independent NCLEX tutor and asking them for help. Your school or a local test-coaching center may be able to provide a name.

In addition, you may want to look into taking an NCLEX review course specifically for graduates who didn't pass the first time. Most of these courses include comprehensive assessments of strengths and weaknesses as well as integrated content review. Some of these courses even have a money-back guarantee if you don't pass the NCLEX on your next attempt.

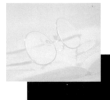

RESOURCES

Web sites

AMAZON.COM ONLINE BOOKSTORE

www.amazon.com

Surf over to the Amazon.com site, type "NCLEX" into the search engine, and—presto—more than 200 entries pop up, rated according to popularity and availability and complete with detailed reader reviews. Make that *very* detailed reviews. Folks feel very strongly about what they like and dislike in NCLEX review materials. Get all the info here before you spend a dime on review stuff.

DR. CARL'S NURSING BOOKSHELF

http://www.nclex-rn.net/

Andreas Carl, MD, is the author of *NCLEX Made Ridiculously Simple* and the developer of this Web site. In addition to information about how to order his book, Dr. Carl includes summaries of other review materials with direct links for purchase. The site also includes a threaded discussion for exchanging ideas about NCLEX preparation.

F. A. DAVIS NCLEX-RN BOOKS AND STUDY HELPS

www.fadavis.com

In addition to the basic question-and-answer-style review books, F. A. Davis Company also has some unique NCLEX review products, including pharmacology, nutrition, and assessment review cards. Use search function to find NCLEX books.

KAPLAN'S NCLEX SITE

www.kaptest.com

Information about studying for the NCLEX is available here. Kaplan also has a number of software review programs available that you can order online, including a diagnostic test on CD-ROM and question-and-answer CDs that simulate testing conditions You can also sign up for a free weekly e-mail newsletter stuffed full of NCLEX study tips.

NATIONAL COUNCIL OF STATE BOARDS OF NURSING NCLEX SITE

www.nclex.com

This site is brought to you by the folks who make up the NCLEX exam, so I guess they ought to be able to tell you how to pass it. This site offers extremely comprehensive online review options for a reasonable price, with 24-hour availability and flexible terms. The site also contains informational links to the NCLEX examination test plan category topics.

NCLEX EXCEL

http://nursing.mcphu.edu/excel/

The site includes review options offered by the National Student Nursing Association in conjunction with MCP-Hahnemann University's continuing education programs. It offers live courses, distance courses, audiotapes, and computerized question-and-answer CDs. You can try a free demo here and even get a free class if you sign up 10 of your classmates.

RN EXPRESS

www.rnexpress.com

This site is operated by Springhouse Corporation, publishers of *Nursing2000 Magazine* and other products, and offers practice tests online for $9.95 each.

CHAPTER 9

Yes, You Can Avoid: Confusion, Chronic, Related to Changing Issues and Trends

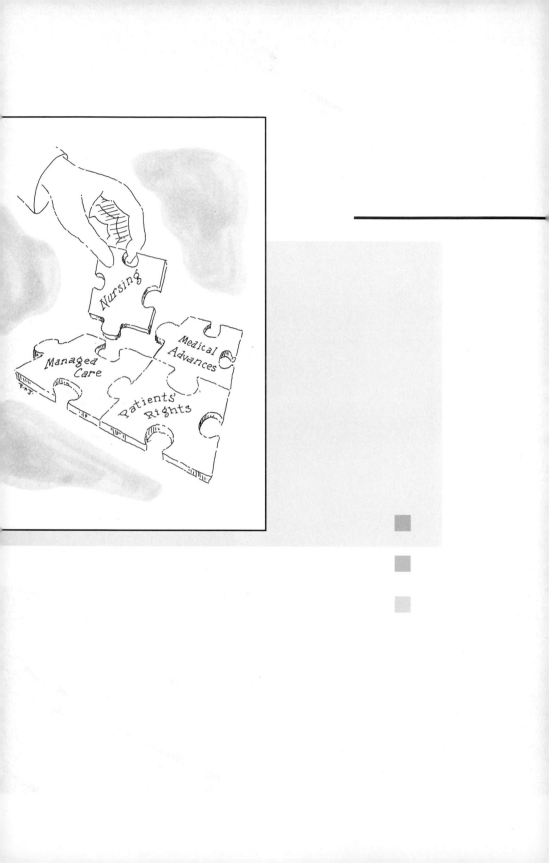

Yes, You Can Avoid: Confusion, Chronic, Related to Changing Issues and Trends

"a student speaks

"I don't get it. Is there a nursing shortage or not? Someone who graduated 2 years ago couldn't find a job even if they had great grades and great contacts. Now, students in the class before us have job offers before they've even passed the NCLEX."

— J.M, BSN student, Washington state

Why this chapter is important

It was Monday morning, just before the nursing center was to open for the day, and I was—once again—whining about writing this chapter. I had spent the weekend working on it and I was—once again—fed up. "No one's going to read it anyway," I grumped to my coworkers. "Ho-hum, issues and trends. This book is for people who are overwhelmed with nursing school as it is. If I add a dry chapter like this, they might stop reading and go back to trying to come up with creative mnemonics for memorizing cranial nerves."

Deb McGrath, a nurse-practitioner at the center, and a faculty member at MCP-Hahnemann University here in Philadelphia, had heard me sing this song one too many times. "Hey, Kelli," she said, over the din of the kids outside who were practicing for their drill team under the window, "get a pen and write this down." I rummaged around in my desk until I found a suitable writing instrument and some scrap paper. Deb continued, "Tell them this is the most important chapter in the book because it gives them context. Tell them that understanding what's really going on in nursing and why it's happening is as important as learning to flush a heparin lock or hang an IV. Many of the difficulties we have had as nursing professionals come from the fact that we tend to treat nursing like a job instead of like a profession. Knowing who we are, where we are going, and what we need to change is what makes the difference."

There were charts to pull and a floor to sweep (we are a very grassroots nursing center) before the patients began coming in, but throughout the day I thought about what Deb had said. I admit I have days, especially when I'm tired or stressed out, when I want nursing to be only a job. I don't want to advocate for my patients, or assess their knowledge or provide teaching, or read up on public health trends, or attend nursing staff committee meetings to argue about collective bargaining tactics. On days like that I just want to give immunizations, cover the kids' playground boo-boos with a Band-Aid or two, write up the charts, and go home to my cat, who's immune to teaching and who couldn't care less if I advocate on her behalf. Enough already. But wait.

If you haven't yet, you will have a class that includes theories and definitions of professional nursing. I'll leave the scholarly discussions for you to have with your classmates and instructors. However, it is important to remember that professional nursing is more than knowing what type of needle to use for an intramuscular injection and whether or not you aspirate when you give heparin. It is more than memorizing facts, being able to quote nursing research, and remembering not to wear patterned undergarments under your white scrubs. These things are all important (your patients do, in fact, want you to know what type of needle to use for an IM), but the key to being a professional nurse is in seeing the whole picture of health care and how nurses fit in.

Learning to surf—keeping on top of the trends

When I was in high school and living in Daytona Beach, we experienced a powerful tropical storm whose name I have forgotten, but we'll call it Harriet. When Tropical Storm Harriet hit the lovely shores of Daytona Beach, two things happened. First, all the surfers quickly donned their wetsuits, grabbed their boards, kissed their mothers goodbye, and headed straight for the water, which was offering some of the best waves Daytona Beach had had in recent memory. Second, unwitting tourists who had parked their recreational vehicles on the beach and were caught by the storm panicked. (In Daytona Beach the sand is very hard packed and vehicles are allowed on the beach. Locals know to high-tail it off when the tide starts to come in.) Some tried to escape the incoming waves by driving on the softer sand farthest away from the water. They promptly became stuck, and many were headlights-deep in the incoming tide before they were rescued. Although I don't think any tourists were lost that day, you can imagine how embarrassing it must have been for them to be rescued by the Coast Guard while sitting in their campers and Airstream trailers. The point of this story is that both the surfers and the RV-driving tourists had a close encounter of the wet kind with Tropical Storm Harriet. The surfers were successful because they knew how to ride the waves and make the best use of the storm. Throughout your nursing career, health care will probably always be in some kind of turmoil. Knowing how to ride the trends and make them work for you will not

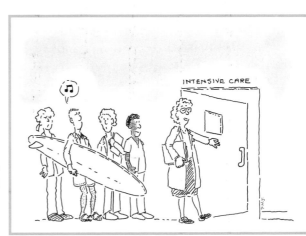

only enable you to be a competent and professional nurse, but also will make the difference between enjoying and succeeding in your chosen profession and merely surviving as a burnt-out nurse.

Nursing in 2001 and beyond: what you can expect

" some former students speak

"Of course, I had a job waiting for me when I got out of school. Honey, I had a scholarship that paid for all my school and even my books, but I had to agree to work in the same hospital [affiliated with my school] for 2 years. I wasn't too terribly fond of that hospital, and every head nurse I talked to kept saying 'come work with us, come work with us.' I had to pick between three very nice offers when I was finally able to move around. It only took me two shakes of a lamb's tail to get out of that first hospital!"

— K.M., Diploma graduate, 1961

"When I graduated from nursing school in 1994, I had worked as an EMT for 6 years, got straight As in all my classes, and had excellent clinical references. I couldn't find a nursing job if my life depended on it . . . which at the time, it seemed like it did. I worked as a unit secretary for 6 months before I finally found a job I hated on an oncology ward. It was a year and half before I found a job I was even close to being happy with."

— **Katrina Dulles, BSN, 1994, New York**

"Everyone I graduated from school with had a job within 6 weeks of passing boards. Everyone! That includes Nancy Nurse (the class brainiac), me (I'm basically a mediocre student), and that guy who sat in the back of the lecture hall and asked really weird questions and always came to clinical smelling like pickles."

— **Jay Roberts, AD, 1996, Pennsylvania**

As you can tell from reading these anecdotes, and as you probably already know from conversations with nurses and your nursing instructors, the job market for RNs is more unpredictable than your eccentric Aunt Jane and more erratic than her driving. And as you can see from the preceding quotes, this erratic job market is nothing new. You only have to pick up your local paper and turn to the classifieds to get a taste of what is going on in your area. Phrases like "Sign on bonuses!", "Twelve weeks paid vacation!", "We'll raise your children!", and "We'll walk your dog!" are all code for "Help, we're desperate!". On the other hand, if the ads say, "Fifteen years' experience required; knowledge of astrophysics helpful" or "Please fax resume and photocopy of latest Nobel Prize-winning research to . . .," you know the job market pendulum is swinging back the other way.

The coming nurse gap

Because of fundamental changes in the health-care system, and especially in how hospital care is financed, the proportion of RNs employed by hospitals has been decreasing every year for almost the past decade. In 1992, 66 percent of all employed RNs worked in hospitals; 3 years later, this had fallen to 60 percent. At the same time, however, nurses are increasing their presence in other settings, such as schools, hospices, home health agencies, long-term care and re-habilitation, and research (Division of Nursing, 1996).

Most experts agree that an RN shortage looms on the not-so-distant horizon. The federal Bureau of Labor Statistics predicts that employment for RNs will grow faster than the average for all U.S. occupations through 2006. Another government study projects that by 2020, the demand for registered nurses will have grown nearly twice as much as the expected increase in the RN work force (National Advisory Council on Nurse Education and Practice, 1996.)

This shortage is building because people are getting older and so is the current pool of available RNs. The average age of RNs began to increase dramatically after 1985 and has increased by 4 months per year since then (National League for Nursing, 1996). Of course, these demographic trends are subject to change because so many issues can influence the demand for nurses. The need for nurses can be affected by such diverse factors as changes in the economy and the health-care industry, congressional appropriations (for example, Medicare and Medicaid cutbacks often lead to layoffs as hospitals try to make ends meet), and, perhaps, random phases of the moon and global warming.

The endangered back rub

One factor that experts find difficult to predict is how many people will choose nursing as a career in the near future. If you have talked

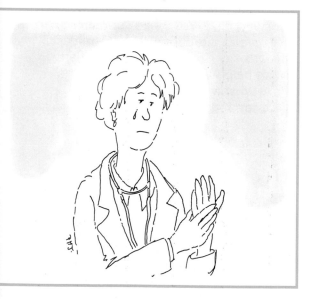

to anyone who graduated from school more than 10 years ago, you know that day-to-day work in hospital nursing has changed dramatically since then. For example, I have a friend who graduated from a diploma school in Kansas in the mid-1970s. She told me that in her first job at a community hospital it wasn't uncommon to give the almost-proverbial back rub to all the folks on her floor before they went to sleep for the night. She said this simple procedure drastically reduced these patients' need for sleep medications.

This is in sharp contrast to an experience I had in 1997. I was in the last semester of my AD program, taking report from the night nurse who had been working with my assigned patient. The patient, who was very sick with breast cancer, was well known on the floor for being demanding, uncooperative, and difficult to please. The night nurse mentioned that the patient had some trouble sleeping, so she used some lotion and "gave her a little back rub"; the patient had fallen asleep and was still sleeping last time she checked. My clinical instructor overheard the report and took me aside afterwards. "See what a difference that nurse made to that patient? It's so different now . . ." She looked down at her hands. When she looked up, I saw that she had tears in her eyes. I didn't realize until that moment how much the changes in patient care have affected nurses, too.

Sicker and quicker and other fast fixes

The most recent changes began in the early 1990s as hospitals were under pressure from all sides to cut costs. Some of this pressure came from decreasing Medicaid and Medicare reimbursements and the costs of providing uncompensated care. Other pressure came from decreased insurance reimbursements, as managed care companies demanded that health-care providers shorten patient length of stay. As smaller community hospitals were driven to bankruptcy by these combined factors and often taken over by for-profit medical conglomerates with headquarters half a continent away, health care became increasingly driven by the bottom line and, frankly, corporate greed.

At the same time hospitals began sending patients home sicker and quicker, they began augmenting staff with unlicensed assistive personnel (UAPs). Although hospitals used nursing assistants in the past to help nurses with some patient-care tasks, the expanded role of UAPs is unprecedented. They are sometimes recruited from among the custodial staff and given minimal in-house training. Some facilities limit their UAPs to helping patients with activities of daily living, making beds, and patient transport. But others allow UAPs to perform more complex clinical tasks, such as monitoring and recording vital signs, checking blood glucose levels, and performing electrocardiograms.

While it certainly doesn't take a degree in endocrinology to monitor a blood glucose level or a PhD to check a blood pressure, the ability to interpret the data is as important as the ability to perform the task itself. In a recent discussion on a general nursing e-mail list I participate in, an experienced nurse described a scenario in which she was supervising a UAP on a medical-surgical floor. When she asked why the UAP had reported a patient with a very low blood sugar level only at the end of the shift, the UAP explained, "Well, I thought it was okay because the patient was sleeping peacefully." The nurse sprinted to the patient's room, where she found the patient in a fairly advanced state of hypoglycemic shock. The UAP was able to assess the blood sugar but didn't know that drowsiness is a sign of possible hypoglycemia.

It is not my intention to personally insult UAPs. Many are hardworking, conscientious individuals who take great pride in their work and in being a part of their health-care team. However, if hospitals continue to use UAPs as they have in the recent past, nurses will continue to have more responsibility for supervising personnel and less responsibility for direct patient care. (How partial are you to back rubs?) If you know that you want to do hospital nursing after you graduate, you should also know that you will be supervising and managing people even while you are a brand-new RN with the ink still drying on your license.

This is both a challenge and an opportunity. (Don't you just hate paragraphs that start like that?) It's challenging because you may be much younger than the other staff members whose work you are supervising, and you may or may not have had any experience in management and delegation. But it's also an opportunity to showcase the leadership skills you developed in your first career as a foreman on a lumberjack crew or in coordinating the daily activities of your spouse and 8 children.

Some BSN programs offer a course in management or leadership; the subject is less common in diploma and AD programs. If you've looked through your school curriculum and do not see such a course, save yourself some anxiety. Sprint, don't walk, to the program coordinator or dean and ask how it can be worked into the schedule somehow. Even a seminar class on delegation or a series of brownbag sessions put on by the alumni association would be better than nothing. If all your fervent pleading and winning smiles don't accomplish any special coverage of this topic, do some self-educating. A good place to start is with a recent NCLEX review book. Most contain questions on delegation, priority setting, and staff placement decision making. Perusing the questions that cover those issues might give you an idea of what parts of this subject you will want to study independently.

The recent changes in health care have affected nurses in other ways. For example, some nurses, especially those who work per diem, have found themselves increasingly subjected to the practice called "floating," or being assigned to work in several different units in the hospital. Although floating has been common for years in some units where the work is similar (such as floating to labor and delivery from the infant nursery), it can lead to unsafe conditions if nurses are required to work in areas in which they are not adequately trained or to which they are not oriented.

What have nurses done in response to these changes? Well, some have done nothing differently and have continued to try to do their job as before, attempting to make up for the increased workload and additional stress by working harder.

Some have tried to cope by working harder and complaining incessantly. If you haven't yet encountered these folks on your clinical rotations, you probably will. While this reaction is certainly understandable, complaining as a long-term coping skill leaves a bit to be desired.

Other nurses have left hospital nursing or are advocating for change within the hospital system. Profiles of nurses who have "surfed" these waves of change and come out healthy, happy, and proud to be nurses are included throughout the book.

Changing the weather

What if you are tired of surfing and want to change the pattern of the waves? Don't laugh—unlike the Daytona Beach tourists, you can make a difference in the changes you see going on around you. When we band together, nurses are a potentially powerful bunch. There are more nurses than any other group of health-care professionals, with more than 2.5 million registered nurses worldwide. Of that number, 83 percent (or 2.1 million) are currently employed as nurses (Division of Nursing, 1996).

Unfortunately, somewhere along the line, activism has gotten a bad rap. Many people (and many nurses) have the idea that activism is not for professionals. They have the perception that activism is for young people—people who don't mind getting arrested, who like to yell at demonstrations, and who wear their hair in spikes glued together with purple paint.

profile

Sylvia Metzler, RN, MSN, CRNP, is an avid gardener and hiker, works as a nurse-practitioner at LaSalle Neighborhood Nursing Center and a primary care clinic operated by Asociación de Puertorriqueños en Marcha (Puerto Ricans on the March), and volunteers at a free clinic one morning a week.

She also recently completed a 10-day sentence at the Philadelphia Industrial Corrections Center, a.k.a. the Philadelphia County Jail.

The sentence was handed down for civil disobedience that Metzler participated in while protesting the death penalty. Metzler was involved in a planned action in which several protesters stepped across a property line while engaged in a demonstration. The action led to their arrest and—they hope—to public attention to their cause. "Of course, civil disobedience is never the first choice of tactics when you're trying to enact social change," Metzler explained. "We talk with elected officials, we have marches and demonstrations, and then if the powers that be still don't listen, nonviolent civil disobedience seems to be the next step in trying to persuade them. This isn't the first time I've engaged in civil disobedience," the grandmother of four says. "Actually, I've been in jail a lot."

To Metzler, providing direct service to people marginalized by our economic and social system goes hand in hand with taking part in direct action to make changes in these systems. "For example," Metzler explains, "as a health-care professional advocating for good health and longevity, I oppose the death penalty because I feel it is sort of the antithesis of that."

In addition to caring about people in her own community, Metzler has a global vision. "I started getting interested in Central America while I was at Yale getting my graduate degree," she explains. "It was the year that Nicaragua received an award from the World Health Organization for its preventative care programs. I went there to visit with a group of health-care providers who all wanted to see the programs that had won the award as well as get an idea of what was happening politically. We spent 2 weeks visiting clinics and hospitals and learning about the country's immunization, nutrition, and breast-feeding campaigns. I was very impressed."

So impressed, in fact, that in 1989 Metzler moved to Nicaragua, where she spent 2 years volunteering at a clinic. She is still involved in the organization Medicines for Nicaragua, regularly traveling back to visit and see how she can be supportive of the country's public health projects and clinics.

Metzler has been honored for her work by *Philadelphia Magazine* and has had articles printed in local newspapers and national magazines and included in a recently published anthology. However, she talks more enthusiastically about her relationships with kids in her neighborhood than any honors or awards she has received.

"For the past 10 years I've chosen to live in North Philadelphia, a community greatly affected by poverty," says Metzler. "It's been a wonderful and disturbing experience; I've learned more than I ever wanted to learn about the privilege that I still have even when I try not to have it. So I've simply been talking and writing about my experience so I can share with other people who have privilege. My goal is for people to understand poverty more instead of blaming the person who is poor for being poor."

Actually, you don't have to dye your hair to do the work of an activist. Activism, after all, means working to change the system in a way that works for you. It might be as simple as writing a letter to the editor or as complex and time consuming as organizing a 3000-person "Nursing Students against Violence" rally.

The most important tool we can use to advocate for our profession, our patients, and ourselves is information. It can be hard to stay informed about current health policy and issues that affect nursing while you're in school working hard to learn to be a nurse, but it's essential. For some easy ways to stay informed see *The informed nurse.*

The Informed Nurse

Or, How to stay informed without losing sleep or driving your family crazy

- Subscribe to the *New York Times* or another daily newspaper with good national coverage. Read it on your commute. If reading bad news that early ruins your day, read it at lunch or just on Sunday.

- Listen to a reputable news radio station while you dress in the morning.

- Watch TV news while you ride your stationary bike or climb on the Stairmaster.

- Take advantage of online "push" features that allow you to access news services. Examples include Netscape or America Online's "news preference" features. You can input key words like "nursing policy" or "health care reform" and have related stories from the Associated Press sent directly into your e-mail in-box where you can read, delete, or ponder at your leisure.

- Subscribe to nursing and other health-care e-mail lists to hear how nurses are handling issues around the nation and the world.

- Join professional organizations, like the National Student Nurse Association or American Nurses Association

- Subscribe to nursing journals like *American Journal of Nursing, RN, Nursing Spectrum,* and *Nursing 2001.* Most have student rates.

"Being nice gets us nowhere"

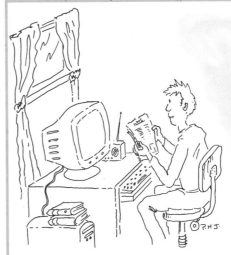

Tho first pooplc wc nccd to advocate for are ourselves. We may somehow have gotten the idea that rolling with the punches and accepting whatever the health-care system and hospital administrators throw our way is somehow an act of selflessness on our parts: suffering so that our patients won't have to. This is baloney, no matter how you slice it. First of all, most of the things we want for ourselves, such as safer working conditions, an end to inappropriate floating, better patient-to-nurse ratios, and appropriate use of UAPs, are things that help us provide better nursing care for our patients. Other issues of concern, such as wages commensurate with the level of responsibility and workload, and an end to mandatory overtime, ultimately affect patient care because a strong wage base and satisfied nurses would mean that more experienced nurses would stay in the profession and provide better care. One well-seasoned nurse activist said it this way: "All we've learned from being nioo for the past 15 years is that being nice gets us nowhere. The answer is not to be mean, but to stand up for ourselves! Just like we have to advocate for our patients, we have to advocate for our profession and for our own health. Far from being selfish, this is the only way our profession will continue."

Perhaps one of the most important, but hardest, acts of activism comes when we simply show up. This can mean showing up to vote in city, state, and national elections; or showing up for those boring committee meetings at your workplace when issues that affect patient care or working conditions are going to be discussed. It can even mean showing up for meetings of your state nurses' association or getting involved with a local chapter of the National Student Nurses Association.

If you are interested in getting involved further, find an issue that really fires you up. There are many issues affecting people's health and well-being that could use a pair or two (or ten) of enthusiastic nursing student hands to help shape public policies. Examples include health-care reform and managed care issues, elder abuse, child abuse, gun violence, and lack of mental health parity (insurers not providing the same coverage for mental health care as they do for other care). Even the ways we use or misuse natural resources can affect public health. You can find information about a sample of organizations that are working to change public policy and educate the public about these concerns in the Resources section at the end of this chapter.

One last note: I am not recommending overextending yourself to attend every committee meeting, political rally, and voter registration drive within 700 miles of your school. The goal is not, in our activist zeal, to improve public health at the expense of our own. However, I have found activism to be empowering. Working with others who share the same concerns reminds you that you're not alone and reinforces the knowledge that others share in the struggle with you.

REFERENCES CITED

Division of Nursing. (March 1996). *Advance Notes from the National Sample Survey of Registered Nurses.* Fact sheet. Washington, DC: U.S Department of Health and Human Services.

National Advisory Council on Nurse Education and Practice. (October 1996). *Report to the Secretary of the Department of Health and Human Services on the Basic Registered Nurse Workforce.* Washington, DC: U.S. Department of Health and Human Services.

National League for Nursing. (1996). *1996 Data Set.* New York: National League for Nursing.

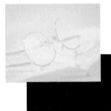

RESOURCES

Books

Bloom, Sandra. (1997). *Creating Sanctuary: Toward the Evolution of Sane Societies.* New York: Routledge

It's an unfortunate fact that no matter where your nursing career takes you, you will undoubtedly work with patients who have been victims of violence. This is an excellent primer on violence and the complexities surrounding our tolerance of it as a culture. Written by a psychiatrist and trauma expert, this book is detailed, fairly easy to read, and surprisingly hopeful.

Gordon, Susan. (1997). *Life Support: Three Nurses on the Front Lines.* Boston: Little, Brown.

A longtime advocate of nursing, Gordon recounts her observations as she follows three nurses through their work at Beth Israel Hospital in Boston. In addition to being a great storyteller, she also manages to sneak in facts and statistics about nursing issues and trends, especially those that deal with how nursing has been changed by managed care. Read this book, and then buy another copy to give to your friends who ask, "Why do you want to be a nurse, anyway?"

Web sites

THE ALLIANCE TO END CHILDHOOD LEAD POISONING

www.aeclp.org

If you are concerned about public health and children, this site may interest you. Lead poisoning is almost 100 percent preventable, whereas the treatment is painful and expensive. It's a perfect issue to interest the budding nursing student activist!

AMERICAN ASSOCIATION OF THE HISTORY OF NURSING

www.aahn.org/calendar

This is a very cool site brought to you by the folks at the American Association of the History of Nursing. It contains a calendar that shows the nursing history for every day. It's great for amazing your classmates with your breathtaking knowledge of nursing trivia and for helping to understand the context of nursing's ongoing struggle for professional recognition and good health for all.

THE CHILDREN'S DEFENSE ORGANIZATION

www.childrensdefense.org

This site is quite comprehensive and contains information on children's health, including information about uninsured children as well as all sort of media backgrounders and a "Getting Involved" section.

CONSUMERS UNION HEALTH CARE INDEX

www.consunion.org/health/health.htm

This site contains many articles, divided into subsections by such topics as health-care affordability, health care for children, managed care, health-care reform, conversions of nonprofit health systems to for-profit systems, Medicare, and medical savings accounts.

DIVERSITY RX

www.diversityrx.org

This site contains tons of information on providing appropriate health care for minority, immigrant, and ethnically diverse communities. It contains information about advocating for these communities and tips you can use to help give patients culturally appropriate health care.

THE FLORENCE PROJECT

www.florenceproject.org

This site states: "We are committed to the providing of high quality health care to all people unrestricted by profit motives, personal attributes, or the nature of any illness." Sounds good to me! It has links to state groups as well as many health-care advocacy links. It also has a very useful "Access the Media" page: If you submit a report of any especially positive or negative media portrayals of nurses you've seen, the Florence Project folks will contact the media outlet from which it originated. The site also includes a frequently updated "Top News" page that links to news features from other sites.

INTERNATIONAL WOMEN'S HEALTH COALITION

www.iwhc.org

Founded in 1980, the International Women's Health Coalition is a nonprofit organization based in New York City that works with individuals and groups in Africa, Asia, and Latin America to promote women's reproductive and sexual health and rights. According to their Web site, they "provide technical, managerial, moral and financial support to reproductive health service providers, advocacy groups and women's organizations in Southern countries."

NATIONAL WOMEN'S HEALTH INFORMATION CENTER

www.4woman.gov

This site calls itself a "one-stop gateway" for women looking for health information. It contains online dictionaries and journals, search features, and frequently updated health news and events.

THE NIGHTINGALE NET

http://geocities.com/CapitolHill/7742/

This site's mission is "to make the face of nursing seen and the voice of nursing heard!" It contains a variety of nursing advocacy information.

PHYSICIANS FOR SOCIAL RESPONSIBILITY

www.psr.org

Yes, I know it says "physicians," not "nurses," but this site is an excellent resource for information about children and violence prevention, as well as nuclear testing and nuclear weapons. It contains statistics as well as information on how you can get involved. It also has a convenient page where you can find your national legislators and, with just a few clicks, send them a personalized e-mail about an issue that is important to you.

Nursing e-mail lists

If you want to learn a lot about nursing in a relatively painless fashion, I highly recommend participating in a nursing e-mail list. For those who aren't familiar with the concept, e-mail lists are online communities, usually set up to discuss a particular topic or concern. An e-mail sent to the address of the list is sent out (via computer or, in some rare cases, manually) to a group of folks who subscribe to the list. Each list has its own individual character. Some lists are full of junk and you have to ply the DELETE key liberally; other are very serious; still others are places where the participants come to know each other well and comment on everything from their socks to their romantic breakups. For more complete explanations and information about mailing lists as well as a more complete description of a number of nursing related lists, see Appendix 2. Two lists that I highly recommend for beginning students are:

NURSENET

http://www.ualberta.ca/~jrnorris/nursenet/nn.html

This is a general nursing e-mail list with more than 600 subscribers from many different countries. Nursenet tends to be a supportive, clinically oriented list, as opposed to some other lists that tend to be rather cerebral and academic. Topics range from how many alcohol swabs should be used when giving an intramuscular injection, to comforting hospitalized relatives, to dealing with verbal violence in the workplace. This is a great place to lurk and listen to nursing wisdom as well as get your questions about the pay scale for new grads in Omaha answered. To subscribe, send an e-mail message to the server at: **listserv@listserv.utoronto.ca**. In the body of the note say ONLY: **sub nursenet Yourfirstname Yourlastname** (e.g., **SUBNURSENET Suzy Scrapple**).

STUDENT NURSE LIST: THE E-MAIL LIST FOR NURSING STUDENTS

http://www.snurse-l.org

I can't say enough about this list. I joined early in my first year of nursing school and couldn't believe what a great community it is (and continues to be). There are folks on the list from New Zealand, Alaska, and Africa. I found it an especially good place to bounce ideas off other students, to get advice about studying for tests, and in general to be encouraged by what folks were doing around me. It helped me realize it was nursing school, not me, that was messed up. This list is very high volume, so don't be afraid to delete when you need to! Recent topics have included the effect of nursing school on relationships; use of humor in working with psychiatric patients; sadistic nursing instructors; and the length of needles to use when giving intramuscular injections to thin eighth graders. To join, send an e-mail message to **listserv SUB SNURSE-L Yourfirstname Yourlastname** (e.g. **SUB SNURSE-L Henrietta Hotcakes**).

Yes, You Can Avoid: Sleep Pattern Disturbance Related to Occupational Worries

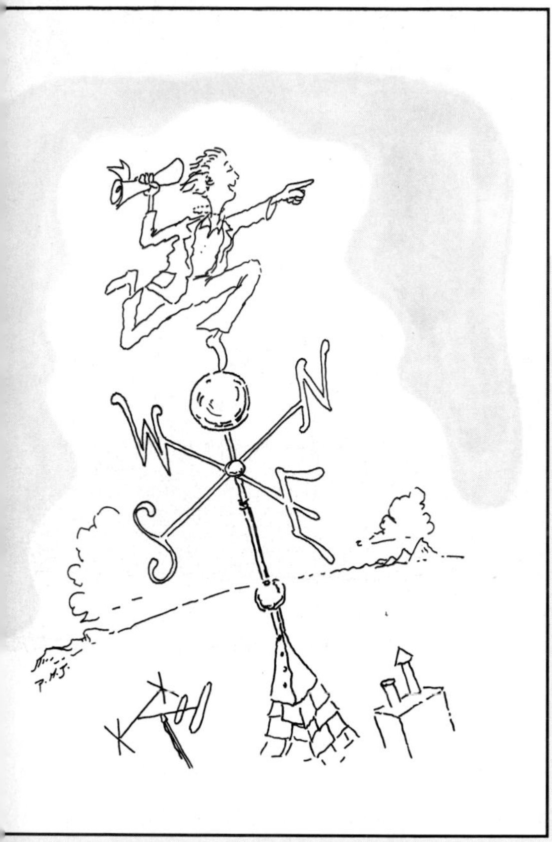
N
W
S
E
P.H.J.

Yes, You Can Avoid: Sleep Pattern Disturbance Related to Occupational Worries

" a student speaks

"I'm trying to be calm, but I can't seem to help occasionally stressing out. I've got one more semester of nursing school. I can see the light at the end of the tunnel. But, even after we graduate we still have the harrowing task of looking for a job. So it feels like the light at the end of the tunnel is really an oncoming train."

— B.D., AD student, Florida

The Job Search, Part I: While You're in School

In a certain sense, all you do throughout nursing school affects your job search at the end of school. Your instructors are the ones from whom you will be requesting recommendations. Folks at your clinical sites are potential future employers. Your classmates are people with whom you will network. Nursing is a very small world. Unless you move to Antarctica to be an occupational nurse for the penguin tenders, you will meet your classmates and clinical instructors in your future years.

You can prepare yourself for your future job hunt by cultivating relationships with your peers, reading professional nursing career magazines, and perusing some of the many excellent nursing career resource Web sites. (I've included a selection of these in the Resources section at the end of this chapter.) Time is tight while you're in school, so if you're reading this on the third day of your second semester, don't have an anxiety attack trying to read each issue of *Nursing Careers Today* between now and graduation. The single best way to prepare for a job after nursing school is to apply yourself to your main occupation while you're still in nursing school—learning how to be a great nurse.

Networking at clinical

In between passing meds, patient teaching, AM care, and trying to avoid annoying your clinical instructor, keep your job-search antennae up while at clinical. Pretend you're an anthropologist trying to figure out how this mysterious culture works; it will be more interesting and less frustrating that way. How do nurses and other healthcare providers interact? How are scheduling decisions made? How do the nurse manager and administrative personnel communicate with, and receive feedback from, the staff nurses?

Observe carefully—even if you are disappointed in a certain clinical site and would not set foot on that floor again even to escape a herd of stampeding elephants. You can learn a lot about what you do want by paying close attention to what you do not want. What exactly is it about the site that you don't like? Is it the way it is managed? The setting? The lack of resources available to the nurses? The outdated patient teaching material? Would you prefer to work with another patient population or in a facility with a nurses' union?

Additionally, you should assume two things about every employee you encounter during your clinical rotation. One is that they have something valuable to teach you, whether it's providing a tip about how to take off adhesive tape without compromising a patient's skin integrity or providing a visual reminder of why it's important to wear white rather than brightly colored undergarments under white nursing garb. The second assumption that you should make is that you will see the person again. Listen to M. L., a BSN grad from Wisconsin: "I did not enjoy my time on the rehab floor during my first semester's clinical rotation. There was nothing wrong with the floor itself, or the nurses, or the leadership; I simply didn't enjoy the nurse's role in that kind of setting. I still did the best I could to demonstrate a positive attitude. I was very glad I made the effort when I interviewed for a staff nurse position on a medical/surgical floor of the same hospital. The nurse manager who did my follow-up interview had recently been transferred from the rehab floor. I got the job, and she was my new boss. I can't say it enough: Nursing is a small world. Never burn any bridges."

Getting stuff for your resume

First of all, put any pack-rat tendencies you have to good use now, while you're in school. Start keeping documentation to support your claim that you will be an outstanding nurse employee. Note every project you've been involved in and every minute you spend doing volunteer work, and keep a copy of every poster presentation you make. Write down detailed information about the duties of every office you hold in any organization, even if it is only being a volunteer assistant to the assistant of your small town's dogcatcher. You won't be able to include all this information in your resume, but it will help jog your memory when the time for resume preparation comes. When nursing school is over, you will be busy doing an elated tap dance on the roof of your house. You can bet that you won't remember that you spent 6 hours taking blood pressures at a community health fair in your first semester of school. Better to write it down when you do it.

Using school resources

Most schools have some kind of career counseling center. This career center can be as uninspiring as a stack of Sunday classifieds in an almost deserted room with no furniture but a vinyl chair with a torn back. Or it can be as helpful as a full-service career center with computers, workshops, and a friendly and knowledgeable staff.

This is the time to really take advantage of the resources your school provides. Don't be shy; you've paid for it with your student activity fees. Bring your sleeping bag and a tent and move yourself right into the career center. Have the staff help you with your resume, get their suggestions for Web sites to check out for job leads, even stop by on the way to your first interview and have them check that your tie is on straight. Remember to get all the printed job-search informational materials you can, and take any aptitude tests they offer.

The job search, part II: getting started

Discovering what's out there

Although much of this book is geared toward students who will be starting their nursing careers working in a hospital, I don't mean to give the impression that this is the only alternative. In a recent advertisement for an informational seminar about career options for nurses, more than 60 different choices were listed. RNs work in outpatient settings, free clinics, schools, factories, pharmaceutical companies, long-term care facilities, homeless shelters, nurse-managed clinics, parishes, insurance companies, and even on cruise ships and at the zoo. Many nurses have started their own businesses; others maintain Web sites; and still others hold political office at the local, state, and federal levels.

You may have gotten some hint of what kind of setting you'd like to work in from one of your clinical rotations, through a nurse whom you personally know, or from a classmate or clinical instructor. To get a better idea about what different types of nurses in different types of settings do, you can conduct informational interviews. Contact someone who has a job you are interested in and ask them if you can interview them about what their functions and responsibilities are.

It's best to schedule these interviews months before you actually start the job-interviewing process in earnest. Be nice, don't overstay your pre-arranged time limit, have your questions prepared in advance, and take copious notes. Take these notes as a courtesy, even if your interviewee is the most boring person ever to set foot on the planet.

It may feel uncomfortable to call a complete stranger and ask them for a half an hour or 45 minutes of their time. But remember that people like to talk about themselves, and when people have particularly challenging jobs, they really like to talk about what they do. Some of the contacts you make through informational interviews may even result in a mentoring relationship. A mentor may be part coach, part guide, part

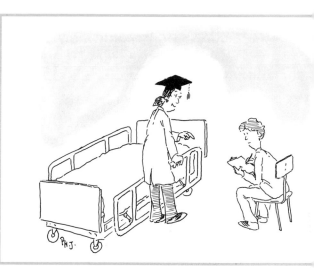

Mentors and Mentees

Mentoring can be a valuable experience for both parties. Here are some tips for making the most of a mentoring relationship

- Be on the lookout for potential mentors everywhere you go in the nursing world. You can find a mentor at your workplace, at clinical sites, at school, during nursing conventions, through the Internet, or where you do volunteer work.

- Be clear about what you want from a mentor. Do you want information about their growth as a professional? Practical advice about the role of a floor nurse? Do you need personal encouragement?

- Discuss up front with your potential mentor the kind of time commitment you are looking for. Do you want weekly phone conversations, e-mail correspondence, or a working lunch every other week?

- Consider what you can contribute to the relationship. Often mentors find that seeing their profession through a new graduate's eyes renews their own passion for nursing. But mentees can also provide other tangible benefits for their mentor. For example, younger grads, especially, may have computer and Internet knowledge that they can share with their mentors.

" a student speaks

"In my last week of clinicals, I mentioned to class-mates that I had been hired to work in an ER, and one of my instructors, overhearing, said, 'Well I don't think that's a good idea because you would be endangering patients.' I replied that I would not have accepted the offer if I had thought so (and I had completed PALS [pediatric advanced life sup-port] and ACLS [advanced cardiac life support] be-fore I started the job). For what it's worth, I had passed the CEN exam less than a year after gradua-tion and now, a little over a year after getting my license, I am scheduled for the CCRN exam."

— **Viane Frye, AD graduate, Florida.**

counselor, and part guru for you as you make your way into the world of nursing. For more information on finding and maintaining a mentoring relationship, see *Mentors and mentees*.

Should I do medical/surgical time?

For many years, some nurse-educators and many nurse-managers have maintained that a new grad is not a nurse until that new grad has completed at least one year working in an inpatient setting on a medical/surgical floor. They claim that the experience allows RNs to develop valuable organizational, technical, and assessment skills, and helps new grads get a firm grip on the RN role and learn leader-ship skills. Pat Reilly, MSN student and nurse-educator at Easton Hospital in Pennsylvania, said, "[The year of medical/surgical experi-ence] is absolutely necessary. I went directly into critical care, but I missed out on a lot of organizational experience. I eventually made up for it but was in a panic whenever I was reassigned." Other nurse-educators' responses to the 1-year medical/surgical floor experience controversy range from calling the idea "poppycock" to saying the experience is "helpful but not mandatory."

Spending a year on the medical/surgical floor is certainly a useful idea, especially if you don't have a clear idea of the type of nursing you're interested in doing or if you feel particularly drawn to medical/surgical nursing—a concentration area in itself. However, the realities of the nursing marketplace are such that new grads cannot always find medical/surgical floor positions even if that is the most desired placement.

Listen carefully to all who give advice about this important decision. Ultimately, however, the decision has to be yours.

When to start looking

" a student speaks

"I'm juggling tests, papers, my job, and my kids. Actually I'm not physically juggling my kids. I'm not that neglectful a mother! But really, I have a million demands on my time. My academic adviser suggested that I start sending out resumes now. Ha! I'm too tired to do anything but maintain."
— **D.R., Second-year AD student, Arizona**

When you actually start answering want ads, sending out resumes, and combing Web sites for openings depends largely on the current employment situation in your area. Some states have an optional GN (graduate nurse) status that allows you to work between the time you've graduated and passed the NCLEX. This license usually allows you to practice in a somewhat limited capacity and most often expires the first time you take the boards. That is, if you fail the first time, you can't work as a GN. You then have to wait until you take the boards again and pass.

Even in states that offer GN status, not all institutions want to hire GNs. Some simply don't want to talk to you until you stand at the door with the wallet-sized copy of your license in hand and a huge smile on your face.

Of course, since you've been sniffing out job leads all through school, a full-scale job search is basically a matter of focusing your efforts. If you hope to work as a GN, you will want to start sending out resumes at the beginning of your last semester. If you can't work as a GN, start researching as many job leads in your area as possible during your last semester. Have your resumes and cover letters stamped and ready to go. The minute you have your license in hand, you can be off and running to the post office, where you will un-doubtedly feel compelled to show complete strangers your license and say, "Look! Look! I'm a registered nurse!"

A resume on resumes

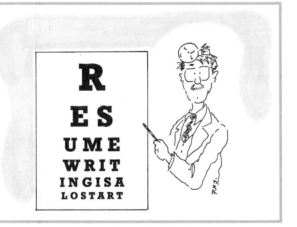

I'm assuming, since you've gotten this far (congratulations, by the way!), that you have some type of resume de-veloped, perhaps from your pre-nursing employ-ment-seeking days. I have included some hints about putting together your resume, but a full re-sume-writing course is beyond the scope of this chapter. If you need more information, you can use some of the many excellent career Web sites listed in the Resources section at the end of this chapter or check your school's career re-source center.

TAKING IT FROM THE TOP: VITAL INFORMATION AND JOB OBJECTIVE

Your resume should begin with your vital information. You should include your full name, address, and phone number. Include a daytime phone number if you can get messages without their being mangled by a malicious voice mail system or broadcast accidentally to curious coworkers. Also include your e-mail address.

The next section of your resume should include your job objective. In phrasing your job objective, talk about how you can assist the potential employer, not how you expect the employer to help you. For example, if you say your job objective is to "gain experience in (whatever)," you give the impression that you are going to be using this job only as a stepping stone to something better. It's no secret that new grads often receive valuable training (both formally and through practical experience) from their first nursing job. However, you have much to offer an employer, not the least of which is your new graduate's enthusiasm. Emphasizing this will make your resume all the more tempting to an employer.

Your job objective should be specific and detailed and about 10 to 15 words long. More details about writing a job objective and examples can be found in the resources listed at the end of this chapter.

Education

After the job objective, list your education and the year you will receive your degree if you haven't received it yet. Spell out each degree acronym, such as "bachelor of science in nursing" rather than "BSN." Most nurse recruiters I talked with advised including your grade-point average if it was over 3.5, but not if you have been out of school and working for more than 12 months. Begin with your most recent degree, and include school names with location (city and state).

Past work experience

List your work experience in reverse chronological order; that is, start with your current or most recent job. Include employer name, location, dates of employment, and a brief description of what you did, using action verbs ("organized," "directed," "completed," "developed," and so on.) To make the resume easier to read, use bullets to emphasize your accomplishments at each job or to outline your responsibilities.

When writing descriptions of your past jobs, emphasize anything that demonstrates how you will make a good nursing employee. For example, let's say you worked at Boards R Us Sawmill in Freezing Falls, Minnesota, for 20 years before you went to nursing school. Let's also say that your job at Boards R Us Sawmill was to fell trees. Granted, there are a very few places to work as a nurse where felling trees would be in your job description, although anything is possible with managed care. However, if you had a near-perfect attendance record at Boards R Us, or if you had an excellent safety record, you would want to emphasize that in your resume since these accomplishments demonstrate desirable traits (dependability, attention to detail) that any employer would be looking for in an employee. One nurse recruiter I talked with said she once had to choose one new grad over another for a single RN opening. Neither applicant had prior experience in health care. The recruiter chose the applicant who had worked her way through nursing school as a waitress. "I figured she would be able to think on her feet, juggle multiple tasks, and understand the importance of customer service," the nurse recruiter said.

If you've never held an outside paying job, or haven't in a very long time, don't fret. You probably still have plenty of relevant experience that will make an employer want to hire you. Volunteer work is the obvious first choice. Again, emphasize projects that required you to work on a team, coordinate activities, and prioritize tasks. If you were ever a Girl Scout cookie mom or a den leader for Boy Scouts, you've developed valuable skills that you can highlight in your resume.

Additionally, it is appropriate for you as a new grad to list clinical experiences in your resume and highlight them in your interview. This is especially important if a particular experience was out of the ordinary or if your clinical experience was in the institution you are applying to. This shows you liked what you saw at the institution, you know what you're in for, and you want to come back.

TIME TO SWEAT THE SMALL STUFF

Before you begin printing out multiple copies of your resume, ask a human who is unrelated to you (and thus relatively unbiased) to proofread your final draft. Ideally, ask another nurse who has a meticulous eye for detail. Don't give a potential employer a handy excuse to round-file your resume.

When you print out your resume, use white or cream-colored heavy bond paper. Use 12-point Times Roman or Arial type font. Your resume should be crisp, focused, and conservative. As unfair as it may be, applicants for Web design or performing arts positions get extra points for using outrageous creativity when they develop their resumes. Nurses most often do not.

COVER LETTERS

Cover letters are usually four paragraphs long and follow a fairly set template. First, mention the position, the organization, how you heard about it, and your current employment status. Make sure to include why you are writing (i.e., the kind of job you're looking for). In the text of your cover letter, talk briefly about your resume, but only to highlight the skills and experience that are most relevant for the potential employer and for the particular position you are applying for. This lets the employer know that you are not only qualified but also interested enough in the organization to have done some outside research about it.

Address your cover letter to a specific person, the spelling of whose name you have double-checked with a phone call. End the letter by providing a phone number where the potential employer can contact you for more information.

The job search, part III: the search itself

Job-search strategies

In order to make the best use of your job-hunting energy and resources, spend some time up front developing a strategy that takes into account your short- and long-term goals as well as prioritizing the aspects of a job that are most important to you. See *The job-search strategy worksheet.*

Once you have completed the job-search strategy worksheet, make a list of potential employers. After doing more extensive research

The Job-Search Strategy Worksheet

Before you begin a job search, write down your answers to the following questions.

- What is my short-term nursing career goal?
- What is my long-term nursing career goal?
- What is my highest employment priority right now?
- What is the minimum I can afford to work for? What is my goal salary?
- Do I have enough information to reach my short-term career goal? Where can I find that information? Is there someone who can help me?

about these employers, you can send out resumes and cover letters that target their potential need for new grads. While you are waiting for replies from these employers, use the classifieds, networking, and the Internet to search out more job leads.

THE CLASSIFIEDS

The jobs advertised through general newspaper classified ads are an extremely small fraction of the nursing jobs available in any region. This is especially true in geographic areas that are covered by regional nursing career magazines. Newspaper classifieds can provide valuable insight into the state of the current nursing job market in your region and can provide some job leads. However, reading and responding to these types of ads should be only the tiniest tip of the job-search iceberg.

NETWORKING

Initial networking can be as simple and relatively painless as telling everyone you know that you are looking for a job. This "everyone" can include your dentist, the person who cuts your hair, your neighbor's cousin's uncle, and even strangers on the bus. I have a friend who got her nursing job because she mentioned to her dental hygien-

profile

"I love my current job: I get to help nurses utilize the Internet in a useful way"

It's 3:47 AM, and Suzy Queue can't sleep. She has a job offer at Quality K Hospital in Punketville, Montana, but she doesn't know how Punketville's cost of living stacks up against the salary offer she's been given. If she wants the job, she has to call the nurse recruiter by 6 AM so she can be on the charter flight to Punketville by 6:45.

Suzy Queue knows she has seen a Web site that compares nurses' salaries in different geographic areas, but she also knows she didn't bookmark it. Where can she begin her search?

If Suzy Queue is like many other Web-savvy nurses, she will turn to *www.allnurses.com,* a popular nursing Web site created and maintained by Brian Short, RN.

Since Short began the site in 1996 (as *wwnurse.com*), it has grown into a full-fledged nursing portal with customizable searching options, sections devoted to career advancement and nursing issues in the news, and one of the most active nursing discussion boards on the Net. If Suzy Queue hadn't wanted to search for Web pages addressing nursing salaries in Montana on her late-night Web sojourn, she could just as easily have joined a discussion about why it's difficult to live with a nurse, exchanged the latest jokes that are going around her unit, gotten career advice, or swapped stories about what ghostly visitors are rumored to hang out around her facility on the night shift.

Short's position as president and CEO of this enterprise, which attracts more than 250,000 visitors each month, makes him a very happy man. "I love my current job," he explains. "I get to help nurses utilize the Internet in a useful way."

Short, a Savage, Minnesota, resident and graduate of Minneapolis Community College, has been an RN for 5 years and held various positions, including working at a nursing home as a staff nurse and a supervisor. Short says the biggest change he has seen in the profession is "[the effect of] cost-cutting measures and understaffing, with a resulting decrease in quality of care that a nurse is able to give."

Still, Short says he wouldn't change anything about the path his nursing career has taken. "If you keep an open mind," he says, "there are so many avenues a nursing degree can take you along. If you get bored or dislike one area, you can always change specialties and have a completely different job." Short adds, "There are ways you can take care of yourself while taking care of patients. Don't fall into the negativity trap, try and keep a positive attitude, and always have a sense of humor, especially with your patients. It will make their day and it will make your job easier."

---

ist that she had just graduated from nursing school and was looking for employment. It was probably no small trick to work her job search into conversation while the dental hygienist had her fingers in my friend's mouth. My friend was rewarded with a job she describes as "more work and fun than anything I had ever imagined."

Your fellow new grads are also a source of potential job leads as well as much needed moral support. One student I talked with suggested that new grads should create a job-hunting club with other members of their graduating class. This sounds like a smashing idea. This same group can provide support through the first year of work while new RNs adapt to their changed role and try to find their way in the professional world.

In addition to in-person networking, I highly recommend getting involved with online communities where nurses gather. Some suggestions are included in the Resources section at the end of this chapter, but a more complete list can be found in Appendix A.

THE INTERNET AND ELECTRONIC COMMUNICATIONS

The Internet has become the tool of choice for many job seekers, particularly in fields such as information technology. But even in less computer-oriented fields such as nursing, electronic resources can be very helpful in the job search.

A rapidly growing number of Internet sites are devoted to helping employers and employees find each other. These sites are particularly useful if you are looking for a job out of your geographic area, because getting a friend who lives in your target area to send you newspaper classifieds can be a major pain. General employment and nursing-specific job sites can be helpful. A sampling of both is included in the Resource section at the end of this chapter.

Most of the larger general employment portals do contain some advertisements for nursing jobs. With these sites, often the most frustrating aspect is picking out RN jobs from the many unrelated healthcare jobs that for some reason pop up when you use "nurse" or "RN" as a keyword. Sites specific to nursing employment are usually more useful. Besides carrying numerous classified ads, these sites offer articles, tips, and tools that can help with your search.

Some sites allow you to send your resume directly to an employer when you see their ad. Others allow you to post resumes on their site or provide a link to your own Web site, which then presumably would have your resume posted on it or contain relevant biographical data. Some sites allow you to post resumes anonymously. If this option is not available, remember that posting your resume always opens up the possibility that your current employer will see it and become aware of your job search sooner than you had planned.

HOME (PAGE) ON THE RANGE

Having a personal home page (a site on the Internet with you as the subject) for seeking employment is to leave the realm of supergeeks and creep into the most technophobic professions. While certainly not essential for seeking a nursing job, having a home page can provide an easy, convenient way for computer-savvy employers to learn more about you and your incredible potential as a nurse.

Even if you don't have a computer at home or don't use an online service yourself, you can still build a home page with one of the free home page services available in every nook and cranny of the Web. Most have user-friendly page editors that don't require you to know HTML (Hyper Text Markup Language, the formatting code Web pages are written in). With many Web page editors, you need only to be able to follow directions and perform simple functions with a mouse to complete your page. For a list of some free Web page services and places where you can get ideas and information on how to make your home page more effective, see the Resources section at the end of this chapter.

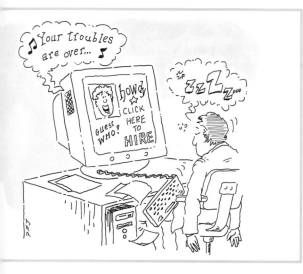

What should you put on your home page? Basically, an employment-seeking home page is an advertisement for you. A resume on the first page is a good start, but you can also post writing samples, a short biographical statement, and even slides of poster presentations you've done for classes or extracurricular activities. You can also include information that you leave off your resume because there isn't room, such as honors or awards.

This home page should be simple and use muted colors and conservative fonts. Use graphics sparingly, if at all, since they dramatically increase the time it takes a page to download. Don't include information about hobbies or other personal activities. Of course, it's reasonable to think that someone can't really get to know you without hearing about your award-winning collection of purple Beanie Babies, but your potential employer may not be so enlightened.

E-MAIL

Even if you don't feel comfortable using the Internet for your search (or don't feel it's necessary), you may find that it is helpful to use e-mail for some aspects of communicating with potential employers. The turnaround for e-mail is usually much quicker than with traditional "snail mail." Using e-mail also saves you the time and expense of buying envelopes, stamps, and paper.

However, e-mail does have its disadvantages. First, the cyberculture demands quicker replies from e-mail than would be expected from snail mail. Potential employers will probably assume that you check your e-mail at least once a day. If your situation is such that you can't check your e-mail this often, it might be better for you not to get involved with e-mail job correspondence at all. Second, the one-dimensional character of e-mail communication makes it easily misunderstood. Each word must be chosen especially carefully, since its meaning cannot be muted or modified by your body language or facial expression.

It's a courtesy as well as a wise choice not to use the e-mail address provided by your current employer to look for another job. Instead, establish a free Web-based e-mail account. Many employment portals offer free accounts, as do most of the sites offering online planner services that were listed in the Resources section of Chapter 3.

Interviewing

PREPARING FOR A SUCCESSFUL INTERVIEW

" a student speaks

"[For a successful job interview] dress nice, cover the tattoos, take out the piercing for now, look people in the eye, think before speaking, talk in complete sentences, smile in the right places, lean forward. That stuff on the 'learned it in kindergarten or from my dog' poster is all-important. Want the job. Act like you care. Do care."
— **Sandra Wolf, MSN student, Wisconsin**

Okay, so between your fantastic cover letter, your sparkling resume, and perhaps even your award-winning Internet home page, you've landed yourself a job interview. Congratulations!

When preparing for the interview, do a reverse reference check. Ask around about the nurse-manager and the administration of the hospital. If the hospital or organization is not well known to you, call ahead and get an annual report and other material from their public relations office. Most large hospitals or health-care systems have a Web site that contains interesting and helpful information about the institution and its philosophy, programs, and clientele.

A few days before your interview, practice your interviewing technique with a friend and do a videotape or practice run at the career center if your school offers these options. This will be especially useful if the center has staff familiar with the nursing job interview process. Practice a good handshake if you don't have one, and ask an honest friend to point out anything you do habitually when you're nervous—for example, pulling at your right earlobe, tapping your foot, or building a tower out of oversized paper clips. This is important because nervous habits can betray your interior distress and distract the interviewer.

Your appearance is especially important. It's helpful to have a navy-blue suit so boring and formal that you wouldn't be caught dead wearing it anywhere but a job interview. Always dress professionally even if you are going in to drop off a resume, because you never know (especially with the current nursing shortage) if you will be asked to interview on the spot.

The backpack you used in school was very practical for lugging around the 2 metric tons worth of texts nursing students carry. However, it gives a slightly more professional appearance to show up at a job interview with a bag that doesn't look as though you might set out off on a wilderness hike at any moment. You don't need to buy an expensive, top-of-the-line elephant-hide briefcase. Instead, borrow a briefcase from someone you graduated from high school with (perhaps the kid who went to business school instead of nursing school) or buy a cheap briefcase to use for now.

When you go to the interview, always bring along an extra copy of your resume and whatever other documentation you have, as well as a pen to write down any questions that pop into your mind during the interview. If you bring an extra pen, you can even loan one to the interviewer if they lose theirs.

In addition to a having your resume with you, you may want to bring a small portfolio of helpful documentation to pull out of your bag, like a magician pulling a rabbit out of a hat (minus the "abracadabra" of course). Items you may want to bring include copies of published articles you've written, synopses of any poster presentations or independent research you've done, copies of your license and diploma, and a word-processed list of three to six personal and professional references. It's very useful to have simple business cards with your name, home address, phone number, and e-mail printed on them. These can usually be made quite cheaply at office supply or copy shops if you buy at least 250 cards. Leftover cards won't go to waste after your job search if you use them to make contacts of a more personal nature.

The day before your interview, call to confirm your appointment time and get directions. Double-check the name of the person with whom you will be interviewing and their office or suite number. Make a trial run to the interview site if you can.

On the day of the interview, allow plenty of extra time to get to the site. If for some incredibly good reason you are going to be late, call the interviewer and explain the situation. If you are detained, maintain a hurried but unruffled composure when you arrive at the interview. Even if you are only 30 seconds late, rushing in panting and out of breath with your skirt askew makes it look like you're 30 minutes late.

ASKING AND ANSWERING QUESTIONS

Job interviews are nerve-wracking experiences. However, the most important thing to remember, as Dr. Roz Seymour, nurse-educator at East Tennessee State University said: "Interview as who you are, not as who you think they want to hire. That way when you become who you are on the job, they and you will not be surprised about whether or not you fit."

Encourage the interviewer to talk by using body language (leaning forward, showing rapt attention, nodding along, and so on) and listen carefully to the interviewer when they question you. It's easy to become prematurely preoccupied with planning your response and miss the whole point of what the interviewer is asking.

When answering questions, be specific and give concrete answers and provide examples whenever you can. This is especially important when the interviewer is asking behavioral questions. For more information on answering these types of questions, see *Answering behavioral questions.*

Finally, remember that you are interviewing the employer as much as they are interviewing you. Always have questions of your own.

Answering Behavioral Questions

When interviewers use behavioral questions, they are looking for a situation in which the interviewee demonstrated particular characteristics or for evidence that they have developed or used a skill the employer is looking for.

A typical behavioral interview question might be: "Can you tell me about a job experience in which you had to speak out against a situation that you thought was unjust?" In this case, the interviewer is trying to ascertain if the applicant is ethical and assertive.

Your answers to this type of question should be concrete, succinct, and detailed. They should portray you in the best possible light. As much as you'll be tempted to break the tension, now is not the time to bring out the humorous stories about your childhood experiences in summer camp. Ideally, use anecdotes from your clinical rotations or past work experience. For example:

Interviewer: Tell me about a time when you used creative problem-solving skills.

Good answer: During my community health rotation, I made a medication instruction chart with pictures on it for a patient who had difficulty reading.

Not as good: Before I had a remote control for my TV, I connected a string to the control knob so I could change channels without getting up from my chair.

One exercise you can do to prepare for behavioral questions in a job interview is to jot down a scenario or two that can be used to illustrate traits an employer might be looking for. If the job you are interviewing for is advertised, you can get ideas from the ad (for example, if the words "flexibility a must" are printed in bold). You can also get ideas from the following list:

What have you done that illustrates that you are:

- Ethical

- Flexible

- Able to think on your feet

- Articulate

- Endowed with good communication skills (written and spoken)

- Willing to go "above and beyond" the call of regular job responsibilities

- Able to maintain flexible but effective boundaries

- Able to deal with stress

- Able to juggle multiple tasks and prioritize

- Able to work on a team

- Able to think critically

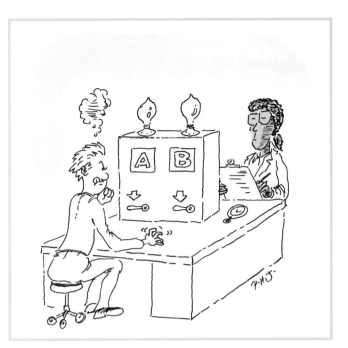

Questions You Can Ask

- What is this institution's philosophy of nursing?

- What type of heath, dental, vision, and life insurance is provided?

- Is malpractice insurance provided? For how much?

- What does your orientation consist of? Could you describe the process?

- Is time allowed for workshops, meetings, and continuing education activity?

- Is reimbursement for tuition available?

- What is the average patient-to-nurse ratio? How are adjustments made for increased or decreased patient acuity?

- Are nurses expected to float to other units?

- Whom do RNs supervise? Are unlicensed assistive personnel employed on the hospital floors? If so, what responsibilities do they have?

- What do you do when a unit is short staffed? When patient census is low?

- How is maternity/family leave handled?

- How is weekend and holiday coverage handled? Do nurses rotate shifts?

Some suggestions of potential questions are included in *Questions you can ask.*

WRAPPING UP

Unless you are Steve Case or Ted Turner, don't expect to discuss salary and benefits at the first interview. Yes, this is unfair, but it is also the generally accepted human resources protocol. Instead, during the final handshake, ask about what the next step is or when you can expect to hear from the employer.

Don't forget to thank the receptionist on the way out. It doesn't hurt to make one little comment that will get you noticed. I suggest nothing far-out like "Well, my trip to Mount Everest was quite nice but when I went to Antarctica . . ." even if it's true. All you want to do is make enough of an impression on the receptionist that they'll remember you if you have to call back to check on the job. Talking about the weather probably won't do it—the last 400 people before you talked about how rainy or sunny it was as they came in. Instead, try commenting briefly on the weather and then talking about the sunrise or sunset the previous day. This is a neutral statement but still adds your distinctive touch.

After the interview, go home and look in the mirror. Tell yourself as sincerely as possible how great you are. Looking for work can be hard work in itself and can make you feel more than a little bit unsure about yourself. Take a bubble bath or go work out or eat brown rice or tofu or whatever you need to do to help yourself feel human again.

A day or two after the interview, send the interviewer a thank-you note. Some career advice folks suggest dropping this note off in person. I personally believe that's too close to "stalking" your potential employer, a practice that will get you noticed but not hired. Send it regular mail instead.

DEALING WITH REJECTION

What happens in the event that you don't get the job? The first thing to do is make another call, schedule another interview, or send off some more resumes right away. If you wait, you'll have more time to brood over the rejection and this will make trying again much harder.

Write a letter thanking the interviewer for their time. This demonstrates that you don't take the rejection personally and keeps you in the employer's mind in the event there are other opportunities.

COMPARING OFFERS

On a brighter note, let's say you've had several promising interviews. You're in demand. The process of comparing job offers is a simple one, but you cannot make the best decision unless you have a clear idea of what's most important to you. A job with excellent salary and benefits is not a bargain if it is located 75 miles from your house and you have to travel by car, bus, pack mule, and personal watercraft to get to work each morning. On the other hand, a job that combines a pitiful salary with a moderate commute and an excellent training and preceptorship program might be a golden opportunity if you are supporting only yourself. A worksheet for job offers is a simple form you can use to weigh each offer based on factors that are important to you. See *Worksheet for job offers.*

Worksheet for job offers

CHARACTERISTIC	CONSIDERATIONS	HOW IMPORTANT IS THIS?
Salary		
Health-care benefits	How much does the plan cover? Are employees required to pay into the plan? Is vision, dental included or available?	
Vacation time	Do employees begin to accrue time immediately?	
Sick time	Do employees begin to accrue time immediately? What provisions are made for short-term disability?	
Tuition reimbursement		
Schedule compatible with other responsibilities	Will you have to rotate shifts? How many weekends and holidays are nurses required to work?	
Proximity to home		
Patient population compatible with desired patient population	Do you want to work in an urban environment? In a small community hospital?	
Specialty area compatible with desired specialty		
Training/precepting programs	How long is orientation? How are preceptors chosen? How committed to precepting new grads is this institution?	

profile

Donna Marie Laino-Curran wears many hats as a school nurse. But the hat she finds most transformative is a multicolored, sequined number with a red tassel on the top. This is Laino-Curran's favorite clown hat, and she finds that it has the power to make even the most uptight, stressed-out Monday-morning worker smile. Clowning is just one of many creative solutions Laino-Curran has developed to address common problems she encounters in the nursing workplace.

"As a new grad working in a pediatric ward on the 3-to-11 shift, I was surprised to learn that at 3:30 PM, after report, the head nurse would lock the toy cabinet and the kids would have nothing else to play with all night," Laino-Curran recalls. "But the thing is, kids like to play with toys. They're kids—that's what they do. When I asked the head nurse her rationale, she said the toys get lost and broken and then there are no toys for the kids to play with. I said, 'Well, isn't that the case now?' So right away I was labeled a troublemaker."

But Laino-Curran thought there must be some way to meet the needs of the kids for meaningful activity after 3 PM. "I went to the library and did some community research. Remember that this was 1977 and there were no VCRs. But we could borrow movie projectors, and so I instituted a weekly night at the movies for patients, families, and friends."

"I never got any praise from the head nurse, but I didn't need it," Laino-Curran recalls. "But I knew what I was doing was having an effect on the kids. Instead of complaining, I found a way that didn't hurt anyone, and in fact it was for the benefit of all." Eventually the hospital was able to get students from a local university who were in the play therapy program to come and do their practicum with the kids in the afternoons.

"It worked out wonderfully," Laino-Curran says. "The students got credit; the kids got to play and also to learn to act out their feelings of anxiety or anger or loneliness about their hospitalization."

It was during these early years of her nursing career that, Laino-Curran said, "My inner clown started to come out. And after my inner clown made an appearance, it became part of my mission to help other folks bring out their inner clown. For example, lots of times I like to use props [when I'm clowning] because it helps to invite people into my persona. If they reach out and touch my [red clown nose] or honk my horn, I invite that. It's a manifestation of the energy I carry around. It's joyful for me when that happens."

Laino-Curran has worked with children in a variety of settings in more than 25 years as a nurse, and she now works as a school nurse in a large urban public school system. She explains that she's not the most conventional of school nurses: "Whenever the kids come to the health room at school, I have them tell me a joke first. This helps to communicate to them that this is an atmosphere in which they can be laid back and it helps them open up to me. The joking also helps to reduce stress for the child and creates a special rapport between the RN and the child. With that rapport comes respect." Laino-Curran paused, then added, "It's amazing—positive reinforcement works so well and yet it seems to be lacking in every discipline I've seen."

In addition to her responsibilities as a school nurse, Laino-Curran is extensively involved in volunteer work both in her own community and in the worldwide community. She has volunteered at the Gesundheit Institute (made famous by the movie *Patch Adams*), has clowned on two continents ("only five more to go"), and regularly volunteers with Habitat for Humanity and Operation Smile. In addition, Laino-Curran, who has adopted two children from Thailand, hopes to establish an orphanage in that country.

Laino-Curran's philosophy of nursing is simple: "I am a healer. All nurses are healers. . . . I wish we could get more comfortable with saying that. I've found that clowns can get away with anything because people feel comfortable around a clown. The whole world is my arena."

Getting up to speed

a student speaks

"As far as self-esteem, I tell my staff (and I do this, too) to keep a notebook handy. Every time someone (a coworker, a supervisor, and especially a patient) tells you what you did right, compliments you, or makes a comment about how well you did a procedure or dealt with a problem, write it down. When you really screw up or make a mistake you feel bad about, tell yourself that it's okay to make a mistake, that everyone makes mistakes and that you learned from this and won't make this one again. Then take a moment to look in your kudos notebook so you can remind yourself of times you were an inspiration to someone else or your being there made a positive difference. It will help you move on."

— Vicki Gustafson, Minneapolis, MN

For the first 3 months of your new job, you may very well do nothing more than come home from work and fall asleep. You will be learning as much as (or more than) you did in nursing school, so be gentle with yourself and keep your support system in place. Develop relationships with other recent graduates in your new place of employment. Even if it's mostly "golden oldies" on your floor or department, you can meet other new grads at in-service trainings, meetings, company functions, or by volunteering for institution-wide committees.

What's next?

Continue to keep yourself aware of trends in nursing employment. You should consider yourself an independent contractor working for your new employer. Never miss out on a chance to upgrade a skill or learn something new.

I hate to mention it just now, but plan to go back to school as soon as you can. When you return to school for your BSN or an advanced practice degree, you may need to work less, and therefore will have a decreased salary, in order to make school possible. The longer you spend at your current salary, the harder it will be to take the cut as you and those that depend on you become quickly accustomed to your increased income level. Even if money isn't an issue, your brain is warmed up and ready to go now, and it's good to take advantage of that momentum.

Finally, feel good about your career choice—and about yourself. You have come down a long, hard path to get to where you are now.

Be proud.

You are a nurse.

RESOURCES

Web sites

ADVANCE FOR NURSES

www.advancefornurses.com

This site includes many ads for nursing openings, all of which are organized into easily searchable categories. If you find a job opening that interests you, you can forward your resume to potential employers via e-mail or create a resume with the site's software by filling out an online form. The site also has career resource links and loads of free articles about writing resumes and cover letters as well as all manner of job-search advice.

THE BEST RESUMES ON THE NET

www.tbrnet.com

Their motto is "no clutter," and they aren't kidding. This site contains thousands of examples of resumes and cover letters and links to other equally helpful resources. No clutter means no long wait to load. Yeah!

CAREER CRAFT

www.careercraft.com

This site features helpful articles.

CAREER PATH

www.careerpath.com

This site contains ads from 90 papers, a significant number of them related to health care. Hit the classifieds without getting ink stains on your uniform.

GREAT NURSE

www.greatnurse.com

This site contains a substantial collection of ads for nursing positions. They monitor their ads closely, so there are few repetitions.

You can also get a free e-mail address (yourname@greatnurse.com) at this site

HOOVER'S ONLINE

www.hoovers.com

Search through 35 job search sites at this one site. Unfortunately, you can search only by state or by rather broad, less than helpful categories. Hoover's does contain more than 15,000 company profiles, so you can do proper research on the folks who are offering you that dream job!

HOSPITAL SOUP

www.hospitalsoup.com

Although not specifically a job-search site, this can be helpful nonetheless. It contains a series titled "A Day in the Life of . . ." (insert nursing specialty here), which is both informative and interesting. The site has some job postings, and you can sign up to get e-mail notification if a job fitting your interests is posted. You can also download patient information educational material here.

THE IDEALIST

www.idealist.org

If you are searching for a job anywhere with a nonprofit community organization, this is the place to visit. It has endless job openings, as well as an e-mail notification service to tell you when a job related to your interests is posted. The site also has some content about working in the nonprofit sector not found anywhere else.

MIRACLE WORKERS

www.miracleworkers.com

This is a job-search site specifically concerned with health care that is fairly easy to search and quick to use. It bars headhunters, so every ad leads to an actual employment opportunity.

MONSTER

www.monster.com

This site contains more than 350,000 job listings organized into broad categories. You can post your resume and make it private or public, with certain information blocked to the public. The site offers resume-writing tips and e-mail alerts. You can also find out how often your resume is viewed by potential employers, if that sort of information is important to you.

NURSE JOBZ

www.nursejobz.com

This is a decent-looking site with a fair number of listings that you can search by specialty area and geographic area. Many of the "openings" are ads placed by headhunters and agencies.

NURSING JOBS ONLINE

www.nursingjobs.org

The list of job openings at this site is rather small, but the openings that are posted contain detailed information. The site is quick and easy to use. You do not have to register to search.

NURSING SPECTRUM

www.nursingspectrum.com

I love this one—it's one of the most comprehensive sites for nursing job-search information on the Net. In addition to sizable collection of ads for open positions, it also contains lots of free articles on resume writing, interviewing, and the like. Don't miss the well-organized threaded discussion boards.

YAHOO CAREERS

www.careers.yahoo.com

You can search for jobs by geographic area, title, function, and keywords here. Typical Yahoo style: easy on the graphics, quick to download. The site posts more than a million job listings at any given time.

A p p e n d i x A

Computers as a helping hand through nursing school

Some common misconceptions

"I'm going to be a psych/ER/veterinary nurse. I don't need to learn how to use computers."

Even if you should somehow find a job that will continue using pen-and-paper documentation forever (home health care with the Amish, perhaps?), you will encounter a computer at some point in your nursing career. Computers are used to obtain patient education materials from Internet sources, to train employees, and to facilitate scheduling and ordering of laboratory tests and even patient meals. Computers are here to stay.

"Nurses are too old/set in their ways/technophobic/ traditional to learn how to use computers effectively."

Older people can learn to use computers as effectively as younger people, and nurses who are technophobic simply haven't been introduced to technology the right way. Systems—especially hospitals systems—that are user-friendly and designed with input from nurses will lead even the most set-in-their-ways nurses to re-examine their views.

"Working with computers isn't nursing."

The corollary of this misconception is that computers are bad for nurses and for the profession in general, since they are (as I actually heard a staff nurse on an oncology floor say) "another piece of machinery coming between us and the patient." The problem, again, is not with the use of computers but with the proper use of computers. Since a computer is an inanimate object—a tool—it cannot by itself be good or bad for patient care. A patient who needs pain medication post-op wants the nurse to use whatever method is fastest to get the pain medication safely to them. The patient doesn't care if the nurse looks up the orders on a Kardex or pulls them up at computer terminal.

Getting started: the very least you need to know

The key to learning what you need to know about computers is understanding that there are many many things you *don't* need to know. You don't need to know how to take apart a computer and put it back together. In fact, thinking more than 7.6 seconds about what's inside your computer is probably a waste of time. You don't need to know any computer programming languages. You don't need to know or care exactly how your computer works. What you do need to know is that there is very little you can do to accidentally harm a computer—at least through the keyboard. So, you don't need to be afraid to try what you want to do on a computer even if you aren't completely sure how to do it. You can take lessons and read books, but the only way you'll ever feel comfortable with any computer is to spend plenty of time with it.

I've included this extremely basic primer for nursing students who have had little exposure to computers. I encourage you to try out the things I am talking about as you read them. Even if you don't have a computer at home, many schools have computer labs, including 24-hour labs, available for students. These labs usually include at least basic word processing and almost always include some kind of Internet access, often with high-speed connections.

First, repeat after me: *"I can learn to harness the power of a computer."* I have a number of coworkers who are as technophobic as anyone, yet when they're left in a room with a computer and a task to do, they are often able to figure out how to do it. Furthermore, there are a slew of happy professionals who are dedicated to making sure the information revolution does not pass people by, and they usually work at the library. You may be able to get informal assis-tance at your school's library, or basic computer classes may even be offered. You can also bribe your friendly neighborhood computer-savvy seventh-grader to give you tips.

Word processing

If you've typed papers or reports on an older electric or manual type-writer, you're going to be dancing a happy jig when you discover the joys of word processing, if you haven't already. Essentially, word processing offers *far more flexibility* than typing for producing final printed projects. The best way to learn word processing, like the best way to get to Carnegie Hall, is to practice, practice, practice. To be-gin, familiarize yourself with one of the more popular programs (Mi-crosoft Word and WordPerfect are two examples) and learn how to use the "help" feature so you can get more information about what you're trying to do at any point while you're trying to do it. Then, volunteer to word-process anything that could benefit from a good word processing. Maybe you have a collection of family recipes penned on stained index cards and passed down from generation to generation. Offer to type the recipes into a word-processing docu-ment, use the "cut-and-paste" option on your-word processing pro-gram to arrange them alphabetically, print them out, laminate them, and store them in a three-ring binder. However, bear in mind that while the program's spell-check can catch some typos and mis-spellings, it won't tell you if the word you've used is the correct word in that context. If you don't follow the spell-check with a close proof-reading of your own, future generations of your family may wonder why Uncle Charlie's recipe for bean soap is stuck in there with all the family soup recipes.

A common fear of people who are doing word processing for the first time is that they will labor over some document for 2 weeks and then "lose" it before it is printed out or saved. This is a natural fear. Who hasn't seen a fellow student at the library or computer lab, sit-ting on the edge of their seat, pulling out handfuls of their own hair, staring at their monitor and mumbling, "I can't believe I lost it" over and over? But thanks to the now-ubiquitous "autosave" feature (whereby the computer program automatically saves your work at preset time intervals), this disaster is much less common than it was even 10 years ago. However, you can still lose a document through various computer malfunctions or if the disk you are saving it to is defective or damaged. Go to an office supply store and buy a few hard-sided containers to protect your disks, and then store these containers away from heat, moisture, and especially magnets (your phone has a magnet in it, so keep phones and disks separate). If you're working on a particularly long or precious document, print out a copy (a paper copy is called a "hard copy") periodically and make a back-up copy of your document on another disk. That way if the computer equivalent of a flesh-eating bacteria destroys your document, you will have a back-up copy with which to re-create it.

To the Internet and beyond

If you haven't been living under a rock or in a subterranean cave, you've probably heard the terms *Internet, World Wide Web, e-mail, usenet, listserv, cyberspace,* and such bandied about. Maybe if you're not online (that's Internet talk for being connected to the Net), you're sick of hearing about it and wish the whole thing would just go away. Well, you should probably save your wishes for a pony or a good grade on the Microbiology final, because the Internet is here to stay. But don't despair—the Internet has a fast learning curve because there is so much to do once you're online, you will hardly notice that you are learning new things all the time.

Browsing around

You don't really need to understand how the Internet works, just how you can make it work for you. The terms *Internet* and *World Wide Web* refer to the network of connected computers that exchange information worldwide. These terms are used interchangeably in conversation, and although there is a technical difference, it's not important to know what that difference is. For our purposes, we'll use the terms *Web* and *Internet* interchangeably, too. It is important to understand that the Internet is not a place; it's the interconnection among computers. When you see something like *www.student-*

nurse.org or *www.scrubsrus.org*, you are being invited to "visit" (i.e., view) a page with this Web site address (also called a URL, or uniform resource locator). The Web page could be located on any connected computer in the world; it's the URL or Web address that tells your browser (the program on your computer that guides you through the Web) where to find the page.

For your first time on the Web, I highly recommend using a computer at your school that is connected to the Internet via a network. You will probably find such a computer in the computer lab or in the library. Explain to a staff member that you are unfamiliar with the Internet and that you would just like to spend some time surfing (that's Web-speak for searching the Web). Bring this book and have some URLs from the Resource sections highlighted that you might like to visit. Ask the staff person, "Where do I type in the URL to go to a specific Web page?" The answer they give you will depend on the kind of Web browser that is loaded onto the computer. Watch carefully when they show you where to type in the URL in case you want to visit another specific URL later.

Once the browser has found the Web page you wanted to visit and has downloaded it, you will see on your screen something that looks a lot like a magazine page. It will probably have some pictures, some white space, and some print. If you move your cursor (pointer) over certain highlighted sections, it will turn into a small hand with its index finger raised. This is called a link, and—miracles of miracles—if you click on it, it will take you to another related part of that Web site or another Web site altogether. This is part of the attraction of the Web; the embedding of links within text (this whole scheme is called "hypertext") gives a multidimensional feel as you click on links and get further and further from where you originally started. And, by clicking on the BACK button on your browser, you can retrace your steps. At this point, just have fun and explore so as to familiarize yourself with the feel of surfing the Web and of using your particular Web browser.

If you surf long enough, you'll find that the Internet has a whole lot of anarchy going on. Unlike more traditional methods of communication, you don't need to have any credentials, contacts, or even knowledge

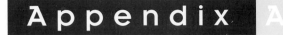
of your subject matter to "publish" on the Web. There is a lot in cyberspace that is interesting and a great deal that is informative, but there is also a lot of cyberjunk. Distinguishing the great from the not-so-great on the Web is mostly common sense and experience, but there are some red flags that you can look for to identify stinker sites.

The good, the bad, and the ugly: Evaluating Web content

Sites that purport to provide health information are abundant on the Net. However, while many are excellent sources, others are useless and some are dangerous. There is no king or queen or president of the Internet, and there are no real binding regulations about accuracy of content. There has been talk of creating an organization that would set minimum standards for Web sites that provide health information. However, the Internet being what it is, adherence to any standards would be on a voluntary basis.

Remember that putting together an attractive Web site requires only computer skills or good Web-site-building software, so even a site that looks professional can be full of errors, omissions, and good old-fashioned fabrications. Fortunately, there are a number of clues you can look for when sleuthing the Internet for reliable information. For example, a reliable site will include the name and credentials of the person writing content or the organization that has developed the content. When quoting results of research, sites should ideally include a full citation for the study as well as a Web link, if applicable. The date the site was last updated should be indicated, as well as the date each article or individual piece of content was posted. Finally and very importantly, on a reliable site, sponsorship or underwriting is either obvious or disclosed. Many sites that may appear at first glance to be informational really are advertorial—the purpose of their content is not to inform but to sell products. This does not mean that all the information on the site is unreliable, only that you should be wary and, if possible, verify the information from another source.

Common Web frustrations

It's not unusual for beginning Internet users to rush to their computer after seeing a Web address while they're out and about, quickly type the address and then hit the RETURN key, only to see an error message that says "404: address not found," instead of the page they were so eager to see. This message simply means that your browser can't find a Web page at the address that you've entered. There are a couple possible reasons for this. Perhaps the Web page no longer exists. Because of the anarchic nature of the Internet, Web sites can come and go quickly, and the 404 message is a detour sign on the information highway. A second possibility is that you have erroneously entered some part of the address while typing it into your browser. With long or complicated URLs, this is easy enough to do, especially when you are getting used to the syntax and parlance of the way Web addresses are put together. Make sure you've entered each part of the address correctly and that you have used the correct keyboard characters indicated in the URL. Common errors include inserting spaces (there are no spaces in Web page addresses), substituting the common endings .htm and .html for each other, and not recognizing that "~" is the tilde, found in the upper-left-hand corner of the keyboard.

Another common reason a Web site doesn't appear when you type in the address is that the server (the large computer at a remote site that stores that particular Web page) is down or not functioning correctly. Servers can go down temporarily for any number of reasons, although extremely high traffic (too many people trying to access the server at once) is the most common. Try the URL again in a few minutes and then a day later.

E-mail, e-mail lists, and "netiquette"

E-mail lists are my favorite part of the cyber-revolution. E-mail lists (also called listservs) are discussion groups in which individuals contribute their 2 cents by composing an e-mail and sending it to a central address (really a computer), which then distributes the e-mail to all the other people on the list. Unlike chat rooms or threaded discussion groups, e-mail lists do not require access to the World-Wide Web, so they are accessible to folks with even the most basic computer setup. Using the Web sites listed in the Resources section of this Appendix, you can find an e-mail list for nearly every topic and interest. If you don't find an e-mail list you like, you can use some of the free services (also listed in the Resource section) and start your own. Some e-mail lists create a very large amount of mail, up to hundreds of e-mails a day. If you are going to join such a list, it's worth it to get a free Web-based e-mail account (you guessed it—there are some listed in the Resources section) to keep your list mail and personal mail separate.

A few words about "netiquette." At the beginning of every semester, it appears that numerous nursing instructors worldwide assign their students to join a nursing e-mail list and research a particular topic. While I appreciate that nursing educators are attempting to bring nursing students into the information age, giving this assignment with no further instructions often causes students to inadvertently wreak some mild chaos on nursing e-mail lists. For example, inevitably at the beginning of each semester, some 20 students join Snurse (a student nurse e-mail list) and immediately send out an e-mail that says, "I am a nursing student at X University. Please tell me three pros and cons of the BSN being entry level for practice." In addition to being annoying, these kinds of posts violate one of the first rules of e-mail list netiquette: *Listen before you post.*

Think of an e-mail list as an ongoing conversation. Would you randomly walk into a conversation at a party and say, "Please give me three pros and cons of the BSN being entry level into practice?" No, you wouldn't, or if you did, your party invitations in the future would be rare indeed. In a conversation, we listen to what is being discussed and get the tenor and flavor of the conversation as well as an idea of what topic is being discussed before we jump in with questions or feedback. If the new subscribers mentioned earlier had done this, they would have found that the Snurse list has had numerous heated discussions about entry-level-to-practice issues and so has made a collective decision not to get involved in further discussions about this particular topic.

The second rule of netiquette is: *Think before you write.* Because individuals engaged in e-mail correspondence don't experience the body language, tone of voice, and facial expressions that can modify or soften our words, e-mail correspondence more easily becomes heated than do face-to-face exchanges. An angry e-mail that is sent out to attack an individual is known as a "flame," and an incident in which a number of heated e-mails are exchanged is known as a "flame war." Before you respond to someone's post on the e-mail list, or any other e-mail, stop for a moment and think, "Would I want this printed out and stuck on my front door?" While it's impolite to forward an e-mail message from someone to a third party without the first party's permission, it happens all the time, and the life of a hastily sent, angry e-mail can be long indeed. It is also important to remember that typing in all capitals is the cyber-equivalent of shouting. As comedian Kate Clinton says, "I guess that means e.e. cummings was whispering. Who knew?"

The third e-mail list guideline is: *Don't send unsolicited junk mail,* especially mail that contains advertisements, to strangers. This is known as "spamming," and it is sure to get a few flames sent your way. The line between spamming and sharing is a bit fuzzy on e-mail lists because, especially on a large list, you are sending e-mail to a number of strangers. If you are selling a relevant service or product and are a frequent contributor to the list, you may be able to get away with an occasional "Hey, don't forget I have NCLEX books for sale on my Web page" post. The key is to contribute meaningfully beyond your ads so that folks will see you as a businessperson, not a spammer. Also in the category of spam are chain letters and forwarded e-mails that contain virus warnings or inaccurate information. While these types of e-mails are always shared in the spirit of helpfulness, they are big-time bandwidth wasters. You will do yourself and everyone you e-mail a favor if you learn the signs of an urban legend (see the Resources section for a helpful Web site). Neither Bill Gates nor AOL gives out money for forwarding e-mails, no hospitals exchange pop tops for dialysis, and there is not an epidemic of injection drug addicts placing HIV-contaminated needles in pay phone change slots (injection drug users have more pressing uses for their time and needles). Only pass on stories you can verify from a reliable source.

The fourth e-mail list participation rule is: *Stay on topic.* Some groups are more vigilant about this than others. Most general-interest nursing groups, for instance, are interested in talking about any health-related topic. In addition, some e-mail lists (such as Snurse, mentioned earlier) provide personal support in addition to

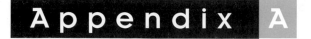

an information exchange. Because of this, a discussion about how much our clinical instructors drive us crazy and a discussion about dealing with teenage kids are both equally welcome.

Finally, when you initially subscribe to an e-mail list, you will be given information about how to unsubscribe. Please, please, please save that message. The same folks who write in the random question about entry level to practice each semester invariably don't save the unsubscribe address and, when they've had enough, send repeated e-mails to the list saying "please unsubscribe me." This doesn't work. It's not that folks on the list are being pigheaded, it's just that they don't have any control over whether you are subscribed or not. Because most e-mail lists are automated, sending a message to the list can't get you off the list. Some groups have tried to avoid this difficulty by inserting a tag line on every e-mail with directions on how to unsubscribe. However, if this isn't the case, and if you didn't keep the e-mail, and if you really must get off the list, pick a goodhearted person on the list, e-mail them individually, and ask them nicely how to unsubscribe.

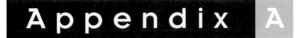

Appendix A

continued

Resources

AMERICAN NURSES INFORMATICS ASSOCIATION

www.ania.org

This site contains job postings as well as information about informatics training and membership in the ANIA.

THE COMPLETE INTERNET SERVICE PROVIDER SITE

www.isps.com

This is a good place to start when you are deciding on an Internet service provider. This site is searchable, illustrated, and has interesting and helpful customer reviews.

DEJA NEWS

www.deja.com

If you have some time on your hands and want to get some really opinionated information about a topic, check out deja.com. Posts to public newsgroups are archived here, so you can read what an expert—or someone who thinks they're an expert—has to say about your topic of choice. Interesting sociologically, if nothing else. Free to use, but you have to register first.

E-GROUPS

www.egroups.com

E-groups recently merged with onelist.com. This site now plays host to thousands of e-mail lists, covering every subject from aardvark choirs to zebra wrestling. Over 500 nursing-related lists are included.

E-MAIL ADDRESSES.COM

www.emailaddresses.com

Calling itself the definitive guide to e-mail addresses on the Web, this site has reviewed listings of almost all the free utilities available in cyberspace. Check in here before you sign up for Web-based e-mail,

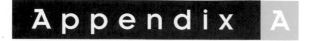

Appendix A

continued

call forwarding, or voicemail services or pick a free domain to host your Web page.

FREE WEB SPACE

www.freewebspace.net/

This site is a guide to the free Web space maze.

GURUNET SOFTWARE

www.Gurunet.com

If you go to this site and download and install their free utility, you can click at many places on any given Web page and the definition of the word or a recent related news item will pop up. It's quite cool—like following a link without leaving the site you're on.

NETLINGO

www.netlingo.com

This site provides a comprehensive lexicon of Netspeak, including an exhaustive guide to emoticons so that you can tell if your coworker is :-> being sarcastic, (:-(very unhappy, or [:-) wearing a Walkman. Go figure.

NURSING SPECTRUM'S RN TECHNICAL SUPPORT

http://nsweb.nursingspectrum.com/RN_support/index.cfm

This site provides threaded discussion with friendly nursefolk who are ready and eager to help you with your computer problems.

THE QUICK METHOD OF EVALUATING INTERNET SITES

www.quick.org.uk/menu.htm

QUICK is an acronym for "Quality Information Checklist"; originally designed for kids, this is an excellent resource for adults unfamiliar with the Web or gullible folks in general. Don't miss the cute cartoon characters that lavishly illustrate the pages.

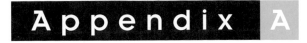

Appendix A

continued

ROD WARD'S NURSING AND HEALTH-CARE RESOURCES ON THE NET

http://nmahp.ac.uk/

This site contains a list of nursing, health-care, and related e-mail groups, arranged alphabetically, with an excellent primer on e-mail lists in general.

TOPICA.COM

www.topica.com

This site provides a fairly comprehensive list of e-mail groups. You can search by keyword or easily understandable categories.

UNIVERSITY OF SOUTH CAROLINA AT BEAUFORT LIBRARY BARE BONES 101: A VERY BASIC WEB-SEARCH TUTORIAL

www.sc.edu/beaufort/library/bones.html

Learn how to search the Web efficiently at this site, which is easy to use and very practical.

Humor for Healing

Even when this book was in its infancy, everyone involved agreed it should be jocular in its approach. We didn't envision that it would necessarily be slap-your-knee, laugh-until-tears-roll-down-your-face funny, but we didn't want it to have a gravely solemn academic tone either. Since this book is about surviving nursing school, it only makes sense that we employ one of the best tactics for surviving tough situations—maintaining a lighthearted outlook.

Maintaining a lighthearted outlook doesn't mean not taking the nursing profession seriously. In fact, the opposite is true. No matter where you work as a nurse, you will deal with humanity in its rawest form, often stripped of pretty smells and social niceties. Whether you're helping out in a code in an urban ER, teaching a 13-year-old to care for their PICC line on an adolescent oncology floor, or leading a discussion on constipation prevention at a local adult day-care center, you are dealing with people where they are, not where we wish they were. As my grandmother used to say, "The drama is already there, child!" Noticing the comedy in the situation only makes our jobs that much easier.

As you may remember from the olden days (i.e., when you started reading this book), I write a humor column for a local weekly paper. Trying to fit the writing between work and school and general life maintenance is often challenging, and there were many times, especially during my first year in nursing school, when I wondered why I was doing the column. The answer came to me one evening as I sat in a diner. I was watching a couple in the next booth have a humorous miscommunication about who was paying the bill, and I scribbled some observations on the back of a napkin that I thought I might use in a column sometime. I had to leave in the middle of their discussion to use the restroom. When I returned, I found that my dinner companion had continued to observe the couple and add her notes to the napkin in my absence. I thanked her and she shrugged.

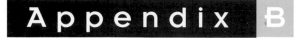
"At first I used to get annoyed when we would go out and you would be scribbling down notes for your column," she said. "I felt like I was socializing with a CIA spy. But now I've started to get into it. I like that you are always looking for funny things around you because now I see more funny things around me too."

Having a lighthearted attitude doesn't mean you have to dress up in a jester suit or clown nose (a la Patch Adams) or start each patient interaction with "A funny thing happened on my way to clinical today . . ." It only means not keeping your nose so tightly pressed against the grindstone that you don't have time to notice the funny things happening around you.

Make me laugh: for you

Besides simply looking for the comedy in everyday situations, you can also create situations in which giggling or guffawing can actually increase your physical and mental health. Humor lends perspective. I used to have a sign next to my bed in my small house in Haiti. "If it's going to be funny in 20 years," it said, "you might as well laugh about it now." When I was able to heed the advice on the sign, it made it easier to spend less time obsessing about the leaking roof and aggressive rats and concentrate more on getting to know my delightful next-door neighbors.

It helps to have a file of cartoons, jokes, and newspaper clippings that make you laugh and pull them out when you're having a particularly bad day. It's nice if your buddies forward you funny e-mail jokes, but don't despair if you don't share a similar sense of humor even with your best friend. One's sense of humor is very individual; my sister literally howls at Woody Allen movies, but I find them depressing. On the other hand, she has no idea what's funny about my all-time favorite TV comedy moment, Mad TV's Gap Troll skit.

You can also use humor as a study aid. You can make up funny mnemonics, write a limerick to help you remember how the blood goes through the heart, or construct a haiku about a difficult-to-remember disease process. One student in a study group in which I

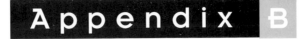

participated set some important information about meconium to a popular 1970s disco tune and would sing it constantly, even while walking through the library. He wasn't so popular with the librarians, but you can bet all the students who hung out with him remember their meconium facts!

Another use of humor is to liven up presentations. You've probably heard your instructors groan about the MTV generation and how no one has an attention span longer than 30 seconds any more. It may be true that music videos and arcade games have left us with few concentration skills. So use that to your advantage. Incorporate relevant (and tame and tasteful) cartoons and pictures into your Powerpoint presentations, or create a mini-puppet theater and write puppet plays about your assigned topic. Your classmates will appreciate the break, and all but the most inflexible instructors will at least admire your originality.

Finally, exercise your play muscles. Think about it: When's the last time you did something just for fun? Playing soccer in a recreational league to force yourself to exercise doesn't count (unless you really love soccer), and neither does attending a business cocktail party as a favor to your spouse. There are lots of fun things to do right around you that don't require much time or money. How about making a paper airplane out of old microbiology notes and seeing how far you can make it fly? Taking 5 minutes to listen—to stop and really listen—to your favorite song or piece of music? Jumping through a sprinkler on your way home from clinical?

Make me laugh: for your patients

In his now-classic book *Anatomy of an Illness*, Norman Cousins asserted that he reached a nearly 100% symptom-free state after he was diagnosed with an immune disorder. He got there through positive thinking and the liberal use of "laugh therapy," such as watching videotapes of Laurel and Hardy and Abbott and Costello movies. Information about the scientific basis of Cousins's claims is available through many of Web sites listed in the Resources section at the end of this appendix.

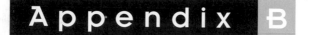
Besides the physiological effects, laughter also has many obvious applications in nurse-patient interactions.

First, sharing a good laugh can help break down the communication barriers between nurse and patient. During our first clinical rotation, a classmate of mine was having a hard time reaching out to his patient's parents, an older couple who had recently emigrated from Hungary. The 22-year-old patient was recovering from a traumatic brain injury, and the parents were clearly distraught but seemed unwilling to talk about what was bothering them. Before lunch, my classmate, who is originally from the Midwest, asked the patient if he would prefer juice or "pop" with his lunch. My classmate saw the horrified expression on the father's face and rephrased the lunch options to "juice or soda?" The patient's father smiled. "I thought you were going to . . .," he trailed off. "Oh," said my classmate, "Give him a pop?" The father and my classmate began to laugh, and the mother and patient soon joined in. Later that afternoon, my classmate was able to talk with the couple about their concerns about their son's hospitalization. A misunderstanding had been turned into a bridge through the power of laughter.

Some useful questions to ask in each initial intake are "What do you enjoy doing?" and "What do you do just for fun?"—and, of course, "What kind of things make you laugh?" Even if you get only a blank stare in response, you will have gathered valuable information about how the patient views fun and recreation. Sometimes we North Americans work so hard at leisure that it is no longer truly a time for relaxation; or, more often, we forget totally about the importance of laughter and fun. When we finally do play, it feels foreign because of its long absence from our life.

Humor can also be a useful tool when working with individuals who feel they must (or naturally do) face illness or injury with minimal outward emotional reaction. Laughing is one way of dealing with the stress and releasing anger about their situation.

There are a number of "laughologists" who have developed tools to use humor for healing, including many nurses. One such "laughologist" is Karyn Buxman, MSN, CSP. You can get more ideas on incor-

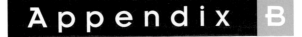
porating humor into your own practice from her weekly e-letter, entitled LyteBytes (see *Lytebytes sample*).

As important as including humor is when dealing with patients, it is equally important to know when levity is inappropriate. Obviously, in the face of an acute crisis humor would be in poor taste. And there are other times when patients need us to be serious. These times might include when a patient is in pain, just after receiving bad news about their health or the health of a loved one, and when a patient meets a new nurse and is not yet convinced of the nurse's competence. Also, individuals in severe psychological distress, such as those with clinical depression, may be discouraged when confronted with a situation that they might have laughed off at one time but cannot deal with now.

Finally, remember that the things that make you and your peers laugh may not be appropriate to say in the presence of patients or perhaps even your clinical instructor. As nurses we need our "gallows humor" to maintain our perspective, but this doesn't mean any patient should hear you refer to any other patient as "circling the drain," "jonesing for Vitamin H," or "in need of a Code Brown."

LyteBytes Sample

LYTEBYTES, WEEK 23, 2000

Welcome to LyteBytes, a weekly electronic bulletin produced as a public service by HUMORx, helping others take advantage of the many benefits of humor and laughter! If this has been forwarded to you, feel free to subscribe using the instructions at the end of this e-zine.

LB SERIOUS LOOK AT HUMOR

H.G. Wells once said, "The crisis of today is the joke of tomorrow." We've all had times when we were embarrassed, upset, even mortified by a situation, only to retell it to someone a week or so later and laugh about it. Humor involves perspective; learning to look at a painful event from a different

LyteBytes Sample (Continued)

angle. It usually requires time, and the amount of time required is different for each person. The next time you find yourself thinking, "Some day we'll laugh about this," try shortening the time frame!

LB FINDING THE HUMOR AROUND YOU

Last week's LB item on the funny sound of "k" inspired a myriad of responses, including the following: "Regarding your recent LyteByte article about the humorousness of the 'k' sound, I must point out an exception to the rule. In the vegetable kingdom, corn is not funny, kale is mildly amusing, and kohlrabi will get a giggle or two. But if you want a sure-fire funny vegetable, you cannot miss with ASPARAGUS . . . and there's not a 'k' sound in it. There is, of course, a 'p.'" (Thanks for those words of wisdom, Dale!)

LB QUOTE

"My greatest fear in life is that no one will remember me after I'm dead."—Some dead guy

LB OBSERVATIONS: BUMPERSTICKERS

If you drink, don't park. Accidents cause people.

Alcohol and calculus don't mix. Never drink and derive.

I took an IQ test and the results were negative.

LB RESOURCE

AATH has requested a call for papers for the 2001 annual meeting to be held in San Diego next January. If anyone would like further information, they can go to http://www.humormatters.com/aathcall2001.htm

For more information about the first national training workshop, "How To Create Therapeutic Laughter and Laughter Clubs," visit http://www.worldlaughtertour.com

LB JOKE

A linguistics professor was lecturing to his class one day. "In English," he said, "a double negative forms a positive. In some languages, though, such

LyteBytes Sample (Continued)

as Russian, a double negative is still a negative. However, there is no language wherein a double positive can form a negative." A voice from the back of the room piped up, "Yeah, right." (Jokes mailer.com)

LB WELCOMES YOUR QUESTIONS AND COMMENTS

CAUTION: LyteBytes is not to be used as a flotation device. Do not submerge in water. May be harmful if swallowed. Newsletter shown is of actual size. No refrigeration required. Discard if seal is broken. LyteBytes is a weekly electronic bulletin produced as a service by HUMORx. LyteBytes is written and compiled by Karyn Buxman, MSN, CSP, a leading national expert who works with organizations that want happy employees and administrators who want their employees to feel better about themselves and their work. The editorial staff has left errors in this newsletter so that our left-brained fans might experience the joy in finding them. Copyright 2000 by HUMORx. To subscribe to the weekly LyteBytes, e-mail to: Join-lytebytes Leave-lytebytes 573-221-9086 FAX 573-221-7226 E-mail Karyn@humorx.com http://www.HUMORx/com

Appendix B

continued

Resources

AMERICAN ASSOCIATION OF THERAPEUTIC HUMOR

www.aath.org

This site contains membership information, conference dates, and loads of links to other therapeutic humor sites.

THE CANCER CLUB

www.cancerclub.com

Christine Clifford founded the Cancer Club after she was diagnosed with breast cancer. Clifford found that during her treatment her family, while supportive, completely stopped making jokes when they were around her. "So Christine began to search for signs of humor in herself and her predicament, and the more she laughed, the stronger she grew." Read more about the Cancer Club and its history and resources on this Web site.

COMEDY CENTRAL NETWORK HOME PAGE

www.comedycentral.com

Comedy Central provided a $75,000 dollar grant to the University of California at Los Angeles to research how to most effectively use humor to reduce pain and prevent disease. Where else can you read about research progress and download sound files from South Park all on one Web site?

CONSTANT SOURCE

www.constantsource.com

This site contains resources from Julia Riley, RN, a well-known speaker and author. Topics include humor in the workplace, team building, managing stress, dealing with anger, and maintaining enthusiasm.

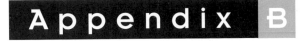

Appendix B

continued

DAVE BARRY AT THE MIAMI HERALD

www.herald.com/tropic/barry

Exploding toilets? Atomic tomatoes? Nope, Dave Barry does not make this stuff up. He's got a nurse's sense of humor, and he's won a Pulitzer Prize for it (much to his consternation). Get a weekly dose of Dave here.

DAVE BARRY COLUMN GENERATOR

www.peacefire.org/staff/bennett/autodave/

Once a week not enough? This site will help you generate a Dave Barry column with just a few clicks of the mouse. Very amusing.

THE HUMOR COLLECTION

http://wreckedhumor.tripod.com/

This site is a gargantuan collection of mostly humorous material, much of it culled from the nooks and crannies of the Internet. Don't miss the canonical lists feature, which includes a list of everything Bart has written on the chalkboard since the TV show *The Simpsons* first aired. My favorite? "Organ transplants are best left to the professionals."

HUMOR RX

www.humorx.com

Sign up here for the free weekly Lytebytes e-letter like the one you saw in *LyteBytes sample* and read articles covering an extremely wide range of humor topics.

JEST FOR THE HEALTH OF IT

www.mother.com/JestHome/

Jest for the Health of It is a company run by Patty Wooten, a nurse, humorist, clown, stand-up comic, and author. This site contains lots of interesting links to articles written by Ms. Wooten for the *Journal of Nursing Jocularity* about the therapeutic effects of humor.

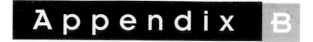

JOHN KINDE'S HUMOR POWER

www.humorpower.com

This site provides free articles and tips about the use of humor for healing and team building. You can also buy audiotapes and videotapes on the same subject.

NURSING MEDIA

www.nursingmedia.org

This site, created by the producers of the musical comedy *Who's Got the Keys?* (think: the keys for the narcotics box), contains information about the show and a great set of links.

NURSING NETWORK HUMOR

www.nursingnetwork.com/humor.htm

A weekly nursing humor newsletter is archived here.

THE ONION NEWSPAPER

www.theonion.com

This is a parody of a newspaper, so don't believe everything you read here. Some of the headlines, however, ring true ("Murder Suspect to Be Tried in Media, Overworked Justice System Glad for the Help").

WEIRD NURSING TALES—THE STUDENTS

www.weirdnursingtales.com/studenttales.htm

I made the mistake of visiting this site while under deadline for this chapter and spent 30 minutes reading it and, literally, laughing out loud. Don't miss the story about what the pharmacist said to the nursing student who needed a 10-mg Coumadin.

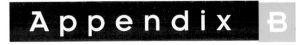

Appendix B

continued

YA GOTTA BE A LITTLE NUTS TO WORK THE NIGHT SHIFT

www.snowcrest.net/lightind/bettyann/limericks2.html

This site houses—strangely enough—a collection of limericks written by nurses (mostly Betty Ann Cassano) about working the night shift. I'm not usually a big limerick fan, but this page is worth checking out.

index

Nursing procedures, for countering unpleasant smells, 159
    process of learning, 149b–150b
Nursing school *See also* Education
    application to, 15–16
    career counseling in, 210
    changes in focus of, 45
    choice of, for gay students, 125–126
    for male students, 128
    competition in, 88–90, 89b
    stress in, 29–51 *See also* Stress
    working during, 62–64
Nursing Spectrum, Website address of, 237
Nursing Spectrum's RN Technical Support, Website address of, 250
Nursing students *See also* Nursing school
    nursing education information from, 8
Nursing trends, 185–205
    activism as, 195–200, 198b
    future expectations in, 190–195
        changes in patient care as, 192–193
        cost cutting as, 193–195
        nurse gap as, 191–192
    importance of, 188–189
    keeping up with, 189–190, 198b
    resources for, 201–204
Nursing uniforms, for clinical rotations, 138–140

Older students, educational program choice and, 1, 4–5, 7
    social factors in, 12
Onelist.com, 66
Onion Newspaper, Website address of, 262
Online bookstores, 23–24
Online courses *See also* Internet
    as educational option, 14–15
    for NCLEX, 176b
Orientation, for clinical rotations, 143–144
Overgeneralization, 35

Paper writing, 90–93
Paperwork, confidentiality and, 157

preclinical, 144–145
Parenthood *See* Family
Patient-nurse relationships, humor and, 255–257
Patients, changes in care of, as nursing trend, 192–193
    in clinical rotations, 156–159
    confidentiality and, 156–157
    privacy and, 157–158, 158b
    nonresponsive, 158b
    as victims of violence, 201
Pell grants, 21
Perkins loans, 21
Personal responsibilities, educational options and, 4–5, 7
Personal statement, in nursing school application, 16
Peterson's College Guides, Website address of, 24–25
Phillips, Jan, 50
Physical resources, in school choice, 14
Physicians for Social Responsibility, Website address of, 201
Play, importance of, 255
    as therapy, 231–232
Practice entry level, educational options and, 3–4
Prelecture reading, 73–75
Preparation, for lectures, 78–81, 80b
Presentations, humor in, 255
Prioritizing, of housework, 119, 120b
    in reading, 75
Privacy, 157–158, 158b
Procrastination, time management and, 60–62
Professional codependence, defined, 37
Professionalism, nursing trends and, 188–189, 198b, 199–200
    in staff-student relationships, 11
Professor Freedman's Math Help Pages, Website address of, 96
Proofreading, of research papers, 92–93
    of resumes, 216–217
Psychosocial needs, of nonresponsive patients, 158b